INTERPRETER OF SHADOWS

Stories of Courage, Compassion, and Inspiration amidst Illness

by Bernard F. Laya

Order this book online at www.trafford.com
or email orders@trafford.com

Most Trafford titles are also available at major online book retailers.

Note for Librarians: A cataloguing record for this book is available from Library
and Archives Canada at www.collectionscanada.ca/amicus/index-e.html

Printed in Victoria, BC, Canada.

ISBN: 978-1-4251-1183-5 (sc)

*We at Trafford believe that it is the responsibility of us all, as both individuals
and corporations, to make choices that are environmentally and socially sound.
You, in turn, are supporting this responsible conduct each time you purchase
a Trafford book, or make use of our publishing services. To find out how you
are helping, please visit www.trafford.com/responsiblepublishing.html*

*Our mission is to efficiently provide the world's finest, most comprehensive book publishing
service, enabling every author to experience success. To find out how to publish your
book, your way, and have it available worldwide, visit us online at www.trafford.com*

Trafford rev. 8/03/2009

Trafford PUBLISHING® www.trafford.com

North America & international
toll-free: 1 888 232 4444 (USA & Canada)
phone: 250 383 6864 ♦ fax: 250 383 6804 ♦ email: info@trafford.com

The United Kingdom & Europe
phone: +44 (0)1865 487 395 ♦ local rate: 0845 230 9601
facsimile: +44 (0)1865 481 507 ♦ email: info.uk@trafford.com

This book is dedicated to my parents, Crispin and Epifania

Contents

INTRODUCTION

"Everything I do is for the benefit of the patients I embrace to care for. I do this for the love of my profession and for the upliftment of my own spirit."

- Joven R. Cuanang, MD

Medicine is a science that is constantly evolving. In the short time that I have been practicing, I have already witnessed tremendous change. More potent medications, increasingly sophisticated machines and more sensitive laboratory tests are constantly being introduced. In addition to conventional therapy, DNA technology and genetics are also being explored. There is a constant need to acquire the best medical technology available, although much of it is used to rule out diseases rather than to enhance health.

Along with these advances, the face of illness continues to evolve. Just as when we think that diseases such as small pox, measles, and mumps have been controlled, more deadly ones come up. Various plagues have come and gone, and every year it seems that there is a different virus causing panic. Hepatitis used to be categorized into Hepatitis A and B. But now, there are types

C, D, E and other serotypes. It would not be surprising that in the future, there would be a hepatitis L. There is also a rise in human immune deficiency virus (HIV) infections, which carry along with them a vast number of co-infections, such as other viruses, bacteria and other organisms yet to be classified. The influenza virus continues to mutate, reinvents itself, and remains a serious health threat. The effects of the previous flu pandemics of 1918, 1957, and 1968 that brought about so much human suffering and devastation, killing millions of people are still fresh in our minds and the current threat of influenza A(H1N1) cannot be ignored. It is also hard to forget the scare brought about by the West Nile virus, Ebola virus, and severe acute respiratory disease syndrome or SARS. Even the number of tuberculosis infections, which at one time we thought was at a declining slope is once again on the rise.

Illness does not only come in the form of infections but also physical trauma, either accidental or non-accidental. There is hardly anyone who does not know somebody suffering from cancer. The more developed our world become, the more we are exposed to things that are potentially harmful to our health. How many times have we heard or read that certain food additives and flavor enhancers are carcinogenic? Still, there are those people whose recklessness placed people's health concerns inferior to their business profitability. Of one important example is adding "melamine" to increase the protein content of milk and milk products. This deceptive ploy has inflicted severe illness to many including the most vulnerable members of our society, our children. There are also illnesses that are congenital, or conditions some people are born with. And lastly, there are illnesses that affect mental health. The degree of illness can be so debilitating that sufferers pose harm to themselves and others. We can't run away from illness. It is perhaps nature's way of maintaining balance, and it will always be a part of human existence.

As the disease process attacks one's physical body, it can also consume that individual's spirit and that of those around him. But inasmuch as it brings physical, mental and spiritual breakdown, illness can also bring out the best in people. It can break bonds and strain relationships, but it can also bridge gaps, reuniting friends and families. Although illness can sometimes ultimately lead to death, to some it signals rebirth and rejuvenation. Sickness can also be viewed as a signal to slow down, and find time for reassessment. It shows us that through courage and determination, there is hope and rehabilitation. No one can escape suffering and pain from illness. Neither does it come announced nor are we given a choice. But when it happens, we have to face it and make the best out of the situation.

Constantly challenged to find ways to deal with illness, we come to rely more and more on machines, tests and pills. But even with the constant advances in medicine, we seem to be always a step behind. We ignore the fact that healing is an active process, taking place in stages, and it cannot be rushed. There is no such thing as a quick fix or "band-aid" medicine. We also forget that physical illness also carries an emotional burden that can be just as devastating. We are constantly in search of the elusive "cure". But there is no pill that treats both the physical and emotional aspects of illness. Laboratory tests, scanners and x-rays can manifest the tangible aspect of disease but it cannot quantify the emotional distress that it carries. This is an aspect of human suffering that is oftentimes neglected. A tumor, a fracture, a disease belongs to someone, not to a "case" or a "medical record number," but to someone's child, brother, sister, mother, father or friend.

Advances in medicine, science and technology will continue, fueled by the changing faces of illness and our desire to eradicate the resultant suffering. The practice of medicine will continue to evolve as it attempts to address the extremes of human conditions of pain and comfort, loss and acceptance, tragedy and recovery, love and hatred. Yet in spite of these changes, only the fundamental principle of healing remains…the concept of one man caring for another, because medicine is as close to love as it is to science.

I am fondly referred to by some of my clinical colleagues as the "Interpreter of Shadows". Indeed as a radiologist, my job is to observe and inspect the shadow images in the x-rays, ultrasound, CT scan, MRI, and other medical imaging tests of patients. Each time I review an x-ray, I inspect the four corners of the film looking at different shadows…the air, the fat, the soft tissue and the bone looking for clues that would fit the patient's symptoms, always making sure to correlate my radiologic findings with the patient's clinical history. Some studies reveal a clear-cut diagnosis but in a lot of patients, I can only give possible diagnosis and some recommendations. Through my observations and interpretations, I become part of the team that initiates the process that attempts to "cure", and eventually "heal" the patient.

But many radiologists are identified only with the equipment they use. Some people believe that the clinician doctors who ordered the imaging study will also interpret the imaging tests. Even worse, some people are not even aware that radiologists are fully trained physicians in their own right. Many people are not aware of the vital role that imaging examinations and the radiologists play in healthcare. There are many diseases that are diagnosed or confirmed with imaging examinations. Majority of patients undergoing surgery usually have at least one imaging study obtained. A patient who goes to the emergency room sometimes feels that the medical work-up is incomplete if an x-ray is not obtained. It is important to note that the radiologist is just as crucial to the treatment team as the nurse, the internist, the pediatrician, the surgeon or other subspecialists of medicine.

Although the bulk of my work includes interpreting routine x-rays to rule out fracture, and looking for source of cough, fever, chest and abdominal pain, I often see devastating pathology. As a radiologist, I am sometimes the first person in the treatment team who sees the pathology confirming the suspicions of the primary physician. Often, I have the task of telling the patients and their families about the devastating news. Many of these patients are already debilitated by their diseases and yet are even more isolated because they don't understand their illness. With the aid of imaging, the radiologist is able to point out the specific abnormality while at the same time explaining it to the patient. The patients and families truly appreciate this because the visual evidence to their illness can help initiate the feeling of acceptance.

As I interpret these shadow images, I am aware that these are extensions of someone else's pain, and each one has a story to tell. In many instances, I try to get to know the patients and take time to listen to their stories. So much suffering arises not just from the illness but also from the feeling of isolation in the midst of pain. People get a sense of real relief when they can share their sorrow with others. Their stories may not be completely connected with the actual illness but it helps unleash some of their burden. We rely too much on equipment and technology, when in fact the diagnosis is often right in front of us if only we would take the time and listen. I have learned so much just by listening and getting to know some of these patients in a totally different way. Each time I sit down with patients and families, I not only become an avenue to provide the "cure," but I also become a part of the "healing" process.

This book is a compilation of stories and experiences. Some are sad and emotionally draining, some are comical and even silly. Some stories can be thought provoking and to others, it may even contradict their beliefs. I have changed the names of the characters and some situations. In some stories, I combined more than one similar situations and experiences. I have done this to preserve and protect the identities of the individuals in the story. Nevertheless, these stories are inspired by real people whose suffering touched many lives around them including myself. Illness has many different faces and in this book, we will meet some of them.

A Daughter Lost And Found

"People love to talk but hate to listen. Listening is not merely not talking, though even that is beyond most of our powers; it means taking a vigorous human interest in what is being told to us. You can listen like a blank wall or like a splendid auditorium where every sound comes back fuller and richer."

- Alice Duer Miller

It was wintertime and the flu season was in high gear, so it took me a little longer than usual to finish reviewing the pile of x-rays from the night before. As soon as I was done, the technologist told me that we had a patient waiting in the fluoroscopy room for ten minutes. This did not stop me from grabbing a doughnut from the office manager's desk and quickly shoved it down, wiping the edges of my mouth as I entered the examination room.

"Good morning, I am the radiologist who will be performing your upper G. I. (gastrointestinal) examination today," I said cheerfully trying to overcome the squeaking sound of the slowly closing door behind me.

"Hello," she responded as she extended her hand and shook mine.

There were several other patients waiting so I proceeded to explain the procedure. The upper G.I. examination is an x-ray test to evaluate the patient's esophagus, stomach and small intestines. For the procedure, the patient drinks barium contrast, a substance visible under x-ray, so that the intestinal tract can be examined. The machine that contains the x-ray is connected to a monitor, so as the patient drinks the barium, the organ of interest can be viewed on the monitor. Della did not appear too surprised to hear about the procedure. Later, I would find out that she had researched it on the Internet several days before.

Della is not the typical patient that we usually have for this procedure. Most of our patients have abdominal pain or chest pain, are vomiting or people who have difficulty swallowing. The study is supposed to find out if there is some sort of blockage or ulcer in the intestinal tract causing the symptoms, but Della has none of these symptoms. She has no problem eating. In fact, she does not only like to eat, she loves to eat. No wonder she is on the heavy side, a morbidly obese woman, and perhaps the largest woman I have ever seen. I did not ask her how heavy she was for fear of embarrassing or offending her. Instead, I walked over to the table where her medical chart was. Looking at the questionnaire, I glanced at the line asking the patient's weight. She had scribbled in black ink, 500 + pounds.

I was worried that our fluoroscopic table could not accommodate her and would break down if I had her lie down on it. This would shut the room down and cause seven other patients to be rescheduled. Since our machine can be positioned upright, I decided to perform the study with Della standing. This way, the machine does not have to support her weight.

"Do you have any questions before we start?" I asked.

"No, none right now, maybe later," she replied hesitantly.

I watched Della get up and walk across the room towards the fluoroscopy machine taking small steps. When she stopped for a second, I asked if she needed some help but she said she could manage. It was painful to watch a lady in her early thirties almost debilitated by weight. I even tried to look the other way because the hospital gown she was wearing was at least two sizes small, thus exposing her backside. I offered to give her a white blanket to wrap it around her waist, but she refused. I was not sure if my gesture was taken as an insult.

"All I needed to see is that you have normal stomach and intestines and that they are in proper place. I don't expect to see any pathology since you don't have any symptoms," I said as she continued to walk towards the machine.

"I sure hope there are no surprises, my surgeon just wants to make sure that my stomach is where it is supposed to be. He said he wants to know the size of my stomach for surgical planning," she explained.

Della is getting ready to have gastric bypass surgery, a radical procedure to help a patient lose weight. The upper G.I. examination is the last test she needed as clearance for her surgery. She is a diabetic with high blood pressure because of her obesity but the symptoms are mild and will not prevent her from having the surgery.

Della drank the barium like a pro not minding its thick, chalky taste. Through the x-ray monitor, I watched the barium outline the esophagus and stomach. Given her very large body frame, I had difficulty seeing the barium as it emptied from the stomach and into the intestines. The large amount of fat draping her abdomen obscured clear visualization of her intestines, so I decided to perform this portion of the study with Della lying down. It would only take a short time and I thought it should not put too much burden on the machine despite her heavy weight. With her lying down, I could at least press on her belly to get a better look at her intestines under x-ray. The maneuver worked and I was able to see Della's normal anatomy on x-ray. I took representative images for her file. Della was thrilled to get a verbal result immediately after the procedure but most of all, she was happy she need not drink anymore of the nasty tasting barium. After the procedure, I shook her hand and wished her good luck before I left the room.

I was in the office helping out with the new pile of emergency room x-rays that needed to be reviewed when the technologist came in and said that the fluoroscopy room was down. This meant that the machine was broken because I pushed it beyond its usual weight capacity. All of a sudden I felt a sudden sense of responsibility for the machine malfunction. I knew that our x-ray table could not accommodate Della's weight but I went through with the procedure anyway.

But our technologist had already rescheduled the non-emergent patients and double-booked the other examination room. "You would have to work faster to accommodate all these patients in one room," Karen, our radiology technologist said with a smile.

Just like that, my apprehension and guilt faded. Karen is a very good technologist not only for her excellent technical skills, but also for the wonderful way she deals with patients and their families especially in stressful situations.

The rest of the morning was uneventful and I unexpectedly finished all the fluoroscopy studies early. I decided to have an early lunch and opted for a quick soup and salad combination. At 11:00 in the morning, the cafeteria was not crowded but as I was about to bring my food back to the office, I heard a familiar voice.

"Doctor, come join me Doctor," a familiar voice called. I knew that the department manager would page me if they needed me right away so I placed my tray on the table and sat across from Della.

"What are you still doing here in the hospital?" I asked just to start a conversation.

"I had some blood tests done," she responded.

I did not push the topic any further because I knew it was an excuse of some sort. There was no cotton ball or a band-aid on either of her arms where the laboratory technicians would usually take blood samples. I was sure she was so hungry. After all, she had to fast for at least eight hours before her x-ray procedure and was now compensating for it. Della did not order breakfast food. She had two double-cheeseburgers, large order of french fries, a bowl of soup, a banana, a slice of cheesecake, and a large soda, indeed it was a meal for at least two people. Della knew she would be undergoing surgery soon but added that she would eat a lot until the night of the procedure knowing that after surgery, she would have to change her eating habits.

Della talked about the doctor who would perform the surgery and how she had decided to have the surgery done. She knew she had to do something about her weight. With her health quickly deteriorating at age 33, she was left with only a few options. Her activities were limited to her work as a filing clerk, working the night shift. She said she watched television a lot, but that surfing the Internet was her life.

"She looks good, Doctor," Della said with excitement in her eyes, referring to a famous singer who underwent the gastric bypass procedure. "They even showed her surgery on the Internet, I watched it. Her preparations, her surgery and recovery, I saw it all on the Internet," she said.

Before that time, I hadn't even thought they showed surgical procedures on the Internet.

"I thought about it for six months and then I researched some more, but one day I woke up and I told myself I am going to do it." Della said.

One could almost feel her passion as she talked. She was so determined to have the procedure done. Patiently, I listened to Della tell her story with so much excitement as if it was her first time telling it to another human being.

Throughout our short conversation, she did not mention any friends or family members and so I asked her if someone would be helping her go through this ordeal. She said her mother would be staying with her during the procedure until she gets better.

"That's great, well if there is anything I can do, don't hesitate to call us, and please stop by after the procedure when you feel better." I needed to get back to the department so I cleaned up my tray getting ready to excuse myself.

Then Della asked, "Doctor, do you have an email address?"

I gave her my business card with my email address, and said good luck one more time before I left.

In the following days and weeks, I became busy. During that time, I was also preparing a lecture on the role of medical imaging in the diagnosis of abdominal abnormalities. I used Della's x-rays from the upper G.I. examination as one of my examples. The fat separated the stomach from the intestines and other abdominal structures making it more distinct, which makes it a good example of what normal anatomy should look like. I also did some research on gastric bypass, and looked up other new surgical innovations in weight loss. It was at this time that I came across the Internet site Della was referring to regarding the famous celebrity whose life has changed for the better, after gastric bypass surgery.

Several weeks later, I received my first email from Della stating how happy she was after the surgery, having lost seventy pounds so far and still counting.

"I am extremely pleased with the results," Della wrote. She was relearning how to eat, taking in fewer meals but with greater frequency. "I listen to my body and stop eating whenever I am full," she continued. She said she now eats for nutrition and to sustain her energy oftentimes reminding herself to eat because a lot of times, she's not even hungry. She wrote about the changes in her appearance and how she felt lighter both physically and emotionally.

For the next few weeks, I got several more emails from Della. She wrote brief notes just to say hi and to update me. She wrote about the time when she went to the park for a walk even though it was cold, when she went to the beauty shop to have her hair done rather than have someone come to her house, and when she went to the supermarket during the daytime rather than late at night.

"It felt so good going to church and seeing all my old friends and neighbors. I used to see some of them once in a while, but I would make excuses that I am in a hurry or act as if I never saw them, that way I would not have to talk to them. I used to feel like I have nothing to share," she recounted in one of her emails when she had gone to church for the first time in 11 years.

She wrote how much fun she had when she spent an evening chatting with a neighbor who had known about her surgery and had been very supportive. But most of all, her excitement was even more apparent when she talked about her first day at work two months after the surgery. Della wrote, "Everyone was so excited to see me. They said I look great. They have posted signs welcoming me back. They even had a food carry in for me. Of course, they had fruits and assorted veggies with fat-free dip." Della also wrote about the time she joined a fitness club to tone up and stay fit. She said she admired people who exercise regularly, something she always wanted to do but felt too ashamed before her surgery.

She also expressed how happy she was to have her mother

take care of her during her recovery. "I made the mistake of distancing myself from my family and friends for no reason other than my appearance. I will never do this again," she wrote. She expressed sadness that her mother had to leave but was excited about the thought of visiting her and the rest of her family in North Carolina at Christmas time.

Although I had not seen her since the surgery, I could picture a totally different Della from the emails that she had been sending me. She was far different from the person I met once at the hospital when she had her examination. She became nothing like the person I had seen at the cafeteria who had to make excuses to justify the amount of food she was eating. It seemed as though the surgery had transformed Della into a totally new person, full of energy, full of life and full of promise.

But the emails have stopped coming after the holidays. I took that to mean Della was getting busier, and meeting new friends so she had less time to spend in front of the computer. She probably was going to the gym much more frequently or maybe she had found a new hobby or even a boyfriend. I imagined that with her job, newly found friends and activities, Della was doing very well. I usually just responded to her emails and never really initiated them, but one time I decided to write her a short note. She did not respond right away, which was unusual. A week passed, and then two, but there was no reply.

One day I got an email from an unknown email address. I was about to delete it but decided to open it when I read the subject; A Thank You Note.

"I am sending this note to everyone in Della's address book.

Thank you very much for supporting Della during the lowest and highest moments of her life. She unexpectedly passed away for unknown reasons two weeks ago when she got back from Christmas vacation. We lost Della once before and it was only recently that she came back, only to leave us again soon after. Prior to her surgery in October, we rarely saw or heard from her. She closed her door to everyone, family and friends alike. She managed to survive independently despite her extreme sadness perhaps brought about by her weight. After surgery, we felt like we had the old Della back, happy, thoughtful, and energetic. She was a wonderful and loving daughter and we miss her terribly. Despite her unexpected passing, we are grateful that even for just a few months we had my daughter back." This email was from Della's mom, Carol.

IT'S A MATTER OF TRUST

"Some patients though conscious that their condition is perilous, recover their health simply through the contentment with the goodness of the physician."

- Hippocrates

One day during my second year of radiology residency training, I came across a familiar name from the stack of computed tomography (CT) scans to be reviewed. Greerdon Wiestock, there could not have been another man with the same name, at least not in Dayton, Ohio. I knew Mr. Wiestock from my other job. At that time, I worked part time as the on call physician at a long-term rehabilitation and psychiatric facility, working nights and weekends catering to immediate and emergent medical needs of the patients. Mr. Wiestock was one of our patients.

I remember one evening when I got a call from a nurse requesting a medication order. "I need an order for Haldol, we have a very combative and agitated patient here on the ward. He is disturbing all the other patients," the nurse said.

"What is he's diagnosis?" I asked.

"He has schizophrenia," she replied.

Since I did not know much about the patient, I decided to go to the ward. It was already 10:00 at night and most of the patients were already in their rooms. There was an old man sitting just outside the nurse's station. I tried to make an eye contact with him as I passed but he looked the other way, he seemed a little agitated but he was not making a scene. I proceeded to go directly inside the nurse's station and briefly looked at his chart to check the medications he was on before I spoke to him.

"Mr. Wiestock, what seems to be the problem?" I asked.

"I just want my toothbrush. Someone stole my toothbrush, I want it back and I need it now!" He replied in a loud commanding tone.

"Well, I don't know who took it but I can give you another one, is that alright?" I asked then immediately told the nurse to bring me a packet of toiletries.

Mr. Wiestock did not respond initially, but as soon as I handed him the packet, which included a toothbrush, toothpaste and a plastic comb, he said thank you and hurriedly went back to his room. I did not have to give him any medication and I did not hear any other outburst from him that evening.

Mr. Wiestock had a CT scan of his abdomen because during his recent medical check-up, his internist, Dr. Patel had felt a lump suspicious for a mass. As I reviewed the CT scan films in front of me, it became readily apparent that Dr. Patel was right. There was a large four-centimeter mass on his right kidney. I immediately called Dr. Patel to discuss the bad news.

"It is the size of a lemon, I suspect it had been growing for some time," I said.

"But he had no complaints," Dr. Patel insisted. "He would complain about the hospital, the staff, his roommate, and the food, but never once has he complained of pain or any urinary symptoms," Dr. Patel lamented almost blaming herself for the delayed diagnosis.

Prior to coming to America in the early eighties, Dr. Patel had already been practicing as an internist in India for several years. Although she was required to repeat a three-year residency in internal medicine that made her eligible to take the specialty board exam in the United States, it was apparent even early on that she is a knowledgeable and competent physician. She had been the internist at the psychiatric facility for nearly eight years, catering not only to the patients, but also the employees of the facility. She is known as a meticulous clinician, and that was why the news about Mr. Wiestock's CT scan findings, of a very large abdominal mass was a shock to her.

I tried to comfort her, "Good thing you found it on your exam. Despite its large size, it does not appear to be causing any urinary blockage problems and that is probably why he is not having any complaints." The brief rationalization seemed to have soothed Dr. Patel a bit.

"I will talk to him today, thank you very much for the call," she said before she hung up.

Bill is a fifty-seven-year-old single male who had been institutionalized for paranoid schizophrenia. He felt people were constantly plotting against him and saw the orderlies, the nurses, the doctors, and even the security officers as enemies. He also thought that members of his own family were possessed by aliens and were responsible for why he was institutionalized. So it was not a surprise to anyone that he did not believe Dr. Patel when she told him about the results of the CT scan, that he had a tumor on his right kidney.

"I am feeling fine. They just want my kidney so they can sell it," he said. He refused to hear any of this and refused any form of intervention or therapy.

One day when I was working at the psychiatric facility, I brought the CT films with me so that I could show them to Mr. Wiestock. I was not sure how he was going to respond but I thought I would give it a try. He was in the activity room where all the patients socialized and watched television. He sat in one corner, staring at the television while mumbling. He may be hearing voices again, as they refer it in psychiatry "responding to internal stimulus." His hands were resting on his lap but they were shaking, a side effect of his medication. I approached him and asked him politely if I could talk to him.

"Mr. Wiestock, can I speak with you in the consultation room?" I asked. He looked at me and did not respond but he got up immediately and followed me to the room.

"Please have a seat," I said while I prepared to show him the image of his CT scan that would show the pathology.

I showed him an image of his normal left kidney and then I showed him an image of his right kidney and pointed out the tumor. I tried to be as simple and direct as I could, not showing him anything else that would confuse him. The whole time I was talking, he offered no response or emotion. Sometimes he would mumble a few words but otherwise he remained seated and silent. I tried to keep eye contact with him but his eyes would wander.

"This is useless," I told myself. I was not even sure if he was paying attention but I continued to tell him what his options were. Then I proceeded to tell him, "You need to have this taken cared of Mr. Wiestock," pointing to the image on the CT scan film, I continued, "this mass is not supposed to be here and it needs to come out. If it gets even bigger, it will cause you a lot of pain, it can even kill you."

The meeting appeared more of a monologue, it felt like talking to a wall. I promised Dr. Patel I would talk to Mr. Weistock and that was what I did. Most likely he won't understand, but then again maybe he would. If I took time and explain x-ray results to my other patients, then surely Mr. Wiestock also deserved it.

The following day, Dr. Patel called. "Doctor, guess what?" she said. "Mr. Wiestock agreed to have the tumor biopsied."

"That is great," I replied.

"He will have it done only if you would do it," she said.

After a brief silence, I said, "Of course, I'll do it. I will talk to my senior radiologist to have it scheduled as soon as possible."

I was really surprised that he agreed to the biopsy procedure because the whole time I was talking to him, I was not even sure if he understood a word I said. I was happy for him but then all of a sudden, I became nervous because although I have seen and assisted on these procedures before, I have never done it by myself.

On the day of the biopsy, I spoke to Mr. Weistock's sister on the phone to get consent for the procedure, she was the decision maker and had the special power of attorney. I explained the benefits and complications of the procedure to her. Soon after, I also talked to Mr. Weistock and gave him a detailed explanation of the procedure. I told him that I was a radiology resident and that I would be performing the procedure, but would be supervised by a senior radiologist. He showed no signs of objection. Once again, he was mumbling words I have never heard before and I felt as if he was having a conversation with himself.

Before I left the room, he said. "Do what you need to do, Doctor." For a second, I had to make sure if the remark came from him. Then he spoke again, "I have total confidence in you." This response was so unexpected because although I was talking to him, I had no idea if he was paying attention to what I was saying. For a resident physician, a vote of encouragement and confidence from patients goes a long way. Although the comment made me feel good, I did not know how to respond to him so I chose not to say anything.

It was ten minutes pass one o'clock in the afternoon when I went to the CT suite for the procedure. Melanie, our CT technologist had already prepared the sterile biopsy equipments neatly organized in a small aluminum table next to the CT scanner. Not too long after I entered the room, Dr. Gregg, the supervisor senior radiologist had also arrived. Mr. Weistock was prone, lying flat on his belly on the CT scan table. As instructed, he remained motionless. The procedure was performed only under local anesthesia. This meant that numbing medicine was injected into his right back area to ease the pain of biopsy but he would remain awake during the whole procedure. I had already cleansed the skin of his back with Betadine and was putting a sterile drape on it when he tried to turn his head.

"No moving Mr. Weistock," I said in a quite irritated tone.

"I just wanted to make sure it was you doing the procedure," he said. An air of confidence replaced my anxiety.

"Do you feel anything sharp here," I asked him while making a small incision on the skin. His non-response meant that the numbing medicine had worked. I then made a small incision at the site of interest. With the aid of the CT scan, the tumor on his right kidney was again localized. With Dr. Gregg confirming my approach, I punctured the skin using the biopsy needle. I did this three times, each time slightly changing the needle placement in order to sample a different area of the tumor. Mr. Wiestock was the perfect patient. This noncompliant, loud and obnoxious old man did not even complain, not even once during the procedure.

"That's it?" he said after I told him we were done.

"We will observe you for a couple hours but you are going home tonight," I said smiling at him as I took off my sterile gloves and surgical gown. He was stable with no signs of bleeding so he was sent back to the Psychiatric facility.

A couple of days later, the result from the biopsy came back: it was renal cell carcinoma, an aggressive and highly malignant cancer. His only option of therapy was to get the tumor out... surgery. Dr. Patel notified me that Mr. Wiestock would have the surgery done only if I was to perform it. Of course this was not an option because I am not a surgeon. But one cannot force therapy on a person especially a surgical procedure. He refused to have any other medical or laboratory tests pertaining to his cancer. But he started taking herbal "tonic" brought by his sister. He took his tonic religiously along with his other medications. But he stood by his decision not to have surgery.

Each time I worked at the facility, I would visit Mr. Weistock. He started to open up to me and to my surprise, he in fact became quite conversant. He told me, "Doctor, I have a good appetite and I sleep well at night. I feel good, I have never felt better."

Although I was happy to hear this, I was still aware that he had cancer. During one of my conversations with him, I told him he was doing so well, but he needed to reconsider his decision regarding the surgery. Then he looked at me and said "I believe I will get better so I am better. I believe the tonic works and so it works."

Then he asked me, "Do you believe surgery will help me?"

"Yes it would," I replied without hesitation. "But I am not a surgeon, you must let the experts do it," I also insisted.

"Doctor, if you feel strongly that I should have the surgery, then I will do it," he said.

After the conversation, I was really astonished and at the same time confused. No one had ever given me such ultimate trust before. I was surprised how lucid our conversation had been, that I almost forgot I was talking to Mr. Weistock. Then before I left, he told me something I would never forget: "I listen to you because you listen to me, and for that I trust you."

Two weeks after my last visit, Mr. Weistock had the surgery done. Despite the size of the mass, it was well encapsulated and the adjacent lymph nodes did not show any sign of tumor spread. This was a good sign. He stayed a few days in the hospital but he was doing so well both physically and mentally that he was allowed to go home with his sister to recuperate. That was the last time I heard about Mr. Weistock.

On the last night I worked at the Psychiatric facility, I had a call to examine a new patient. The police brought in a forty-five-year-old manic-depressive black female who had been wandering the streets downtown yelling profanities. She was unkept and disheveled.

"This one is a hopeless case, Doc," the arresting officer claimed as he uncuffed the patient. "She has been in and out of this facility, a frequent flyer," he continued.

Ignoring the officer's remarks, I asked the nurses to bathe her and give her clean clothes. In my mind I said to myself, "She will come around, she will surprise us all one day."

THE RED STICKER

"The most important thing in illness is never to lose heart."

> -   - Nikolai Lenin

Dr. Michael Ward is one of the more senior physicians at a small private hospital in Southern California where I was doing my medical internship. At six feet and two inches tall, he was easily recognizable whenever he was present in any gathering. He had a very distinguished look with a full set of neatly combed, salt and pepper colored hair, complemented by a well-trimmed mustache. He always wore a long white doctor's coat but one could recognize that he paid attention to his attire, his necktie and pants of the same color every time. He spoke with baritone voice that although monotonous still managed to keep people's attention. At the time of my Internship, Dr. Ward was fifty-nine-years-old but had no plans of retiring any time soon. He was a member of the hospital board and the Chairman of the department of internal medicine. He had an active hospital practice as the consultant infectious disease specialist, and he had a busy outpatient clinic.

Dr. Ward's office is in the Professional Staff building across the street from the hospital. I had already done a couple of outpatient rotations and I felt quite confident when seeing patients. Dr. Ward's patients were mostly routine, redundant cases of high blood pressure, diabetes, high cholesterol, cough and cold and some other minor problems that I had dealt with before. During my first week, I just followed him around as he saw his patients but the following week, he assigned specific patients for me to see. I would first review the patient's chart before I saw the patient and got their clinical history. After this, I would step out of the examination room; formulate the problem list, and outline the method of possible intervention before I presented them to Dr. Ward. If it was a non-complicated patient and he agreed with the way I handled the history-taking, examination, and plan of action, he would just sign the medication prescription that I had already prepared for the patient.

It was my third week working with Dr. Ward and I thought he had already developed a sense of trust in me. Dr. Ward is an excellent teacher, very patient and considerate. At the end of each day, we would usually sit in his office as he reviewed the charts of all the patients we had seen that day. This was when I got to ask him questions, especially regarding the medical management of the patients. This was also the time when he would usually ask me questions about the reading assignment he gave me the previous day.

Most days, Dr. Ward had a steady flow of patients but it was never too overwhelming. I guess I was lucky to rotate with him during fall, before the flu season. One afternoon was unusually slow. It was already 3:30 PM and I had seen only two patients since I came back from lunch. I was at the reception desk area chatting with the nurses and receptionist when a patient walked in. She was a tall and slender Caucasian lady with straight, shoulder length platinum blonde hair. Her prominent nose stood out in her heavily made up face. She wore a flowing silk red dress with length just below her knees. She had on a string of pink pearl necklace complemented by a set of pearl earrings. She was not the typical patient that we see in Dr. Ward's clinic. She looked like she was going out for a party rather than see a doctor.

"Good afternoon Miss Ava," the receptionist greeted the patient. Miss Ava smiled but she did not say much. She was then ushered to examination room number 1 for the nurse to take her blood pressure, pulse and temperature. I waited until the nurse was done taking the patient's vital signs but when the nurse got out of the room she yelled, "Dr. Ward, patient is ready in room 1."

The nurse realized I was already standing by the door waiting to see the patient but then she said, "Red sticker on the medical chart." She was pointing to a large tag taped at the cover of Miss Ava's medical chart, then she continued, " it means Ava is a private patient of Dr. Ward, it also means no medical students, interns or residents allowed."

"Oh I see, one of those, I probably would not want to be attended to by a medical student or an intern if I was seeing a doctor myself," I jokingly said.

Dr. Ward entered examination room 1 carrying the very thick medical chart that was handed to him by the nurse. This patient must have seen Dr. Ward quite a few times and I wondered what her complaint was, but if she was too sick, at least she did not look like she was.

Before I had a chance to ask the nurse about Ava who seems to be known by everyone in the office, I was handed a chart of another patient who had just walked in. The patient was an obese, seventy-year-old female, a smoker with high blood pressure, diabetes, heart disease and depression.

"This is going to be a long one," the nurse said.

"Oh I know it would be," I replied.

Mrs. Jones was my last patient of the day. It was an exhausting task looking thru her medical chart and reviewing the list of her medications to make sure none of them were aggravating her various medical conditions. Afterwards, I spoke to Dr. Ward about Mrs. Jones.

"Everything is good, I am glad you checked and double checked everything," Dr. Ward confidently said. "Mrs. Jones is doing wonderful, continue her medications."

When I spoke to the nurse afterwards, I realized Mrs. Jones had just come in to have her yearly blood work done. A bit embarrassed, I told myself at least I had gotten to know Mrs. Jones.

Several weeks later, I finished my outpatient rotations and was doing mostly hospital rotations. That month, I was at the intensive care unit (ICU) for a much different rotation. It was faster paced, more demanding both academically and physically. There was certainly a higher degree of stress level. In the ICU, patients are very sick and demand closer observation. There were many times at night when we were woken up to give and adjust medications, order and check blood tests, and to perform other interventions. It was not uncommon to get woken up by a "code", meaning someone had had a cardiac arrest and needed resuscitation. It was also during my ICU rotation that I got a lot of exposure talking to the families of very sick patients.

I started my usual routine of visiting each patient during my rounds, performing quick physical assessments and then checking their laboratory tests and vital signs. I was already writing my notes at the nurse's station when I was interrupted by one of the nurses.

"There is a new patient waiting to be transported to ICU," she said.

"What is the diagnosis," I asked.

"Sepsis and dehydration," she quickly replied.

"The patient is still in the radiology department getting x-rays but is definitely coming here," said the other nurse.

I continued writing my notes when the nurse interrupted me again, "By the way, don't worry about the next patient, the chart has a red sticker on it, Dr. Ward will take care of it, a direct admit from his office."

I was pleased to hear the news, at least I didn't have to rush and see the patient. Having four very sick patients on my service was stressful enough.

It was during internship that I realized I wanted to become a radiologist, so I made it a point to habitually visit the radiology department and check the x-rays of the patients in the ICU. One by one I checked my list. Katherine Wilson had a CT scan of her head. She had had a massive stroke involving the right side of her brain. Of course at that time, I could not have come up with that interpretation on my own. I needed to read the final report of the radiologist, which said: infarction involving the distribution of the right middle cerebral artery. Mr. Mendez had a follow up abdominal x-ray, he was diagnosed with pancreatitis, an inflammation of the pancreas related perhaps to his alcoholism. I compared the new x-ray from his old one a week before. "The intestinal distention is getting better," I told the medical student with me at that time. This finding I thought I was confident enough to make but I still peeked at the radiologist's report. Then we checked Mrs. Smith's chest x-ray. She had suffered a heart attack that resulted in pulmonary edema, the pumping action of her heart weakened and caused fluid to leak and accumulate in her lungs. She had been in the ICU for a week and she was showing great progress. Her chest x-ray was also much improved.

"How about Roger Stamp," the medical student said.

"Well we don't really need to check on him, Dr. Ward will be taking care of him directly," I said.

Before I could say another word, the medical student had gotten a hold of his x-ray films. Also interested in how it looked, I took the x-rays out and hung it on the viewbox. I checked the label to make sure I was looking at the right x-ray. For a thirty-one-year-old man, his lungs looked awful. On the right upper lung, there was significant abnormality with calcifications, cavities and significant scarring.

"I know what this is, this is tuberculosis, this patient has tuberculosis," I said. "No wonder they don't want any residents or students," I rationalized. At that time, I made up my mind to see Roger Stamp. All I have to do is wear a gown, a mask and glove up, there was nothing to it. I was not afraid, I had seen tuberculosis patients before.

Tina, the nurse paged Dr. Ward two times but he did not call back. The patient in room 3 wanted something for severe nausea.

"I could see him Tina, I have time, I have already seen the other patients," I politely offered.

"Well, the chart says no interns or students…sorry," the ICU nurse declined my offer, giving me a mischievous grin before she walked away.

What if he is in severe distress, I said to myself, he would still be my responsibility. So I made a decision, I was going to see Mr. Stamp. I put on a hospital gown, a mask, and a pair of gloves before I proceeded to ICU room 3, rolled open the sliding glass door and adjusted the curtain. Mr. Stamp's entire body was covered with a blanket, only his head was exposed. He was lying on his side facing the window opposite me and I could only see the back of his head.

"Good morning Mr. Stamp," I greeted him.

"Go away, you are not Dr. Ward, I don't need anything from you," he replied rather irritated.

"Well, you need medication don't you?" I asked.

"Are you the nurse?" he rhetorically responded.

"No I am the intern here in ICU this month," I responded.

Then he turned over and looked at me. He had long blonde hair and feminine facial features that looked familiar to me. I knew I had seen him before but I could not remember when or where.

"And why are you dressed like that?" Mr. Stamp asked.

"Well just standard precaution for all patients with tuberculosis," I said.

"Get out of here, If you are to see me you should at least have the decency to read my medical record," he said.

I had never been embarrassed by a patient before, the way I was by Mr. Stamp. I really had nothing much to say so I stepped out of the room, and took the gown, the glove and the mask off. I was just glad there were no medical students with me at the time to witness the embarrassing moment, a doctor basically thrown out of the patient's room by the patient himself.

Although this was the first time I was yelled at by a patient, being yelled at as an intern is not necessarily a unique situation. As a young intern, I got yelled at by all sorts of people, by the nurses, doctors, people from the medical educations office and at one time by the janitor for stepping on a recently mopped floor. So I was used to it. I proceeded to the nursing station to read Mr. Stamp's medical chart when nurse Tina saw me.

"So, Ava gave you the attitude?" the nurse said smiling.

"Ava?" I paused for a second before it hit me. I knew I recognized his face. Mr. Roger Stamp is Ava.

The admitting clinical history stated "Thirty one year old Caucasian male transvestite admitted for severe dehydration from nausea, vomiting and diarrhea. The patient was diagnosed with HIV two years ago and now has a very low T-cell count. His weak immune system makes him susceptible to other opportunistic infections. The patient had tuberculosis infection a year ago that was treated." As his impression, Dr. Ward thought that Ava's diarrhea and vomiting are due to opportunistic infections. I felt rather stupid to think that Ava had active tuberculosis. He was not even coughing. That experience taught me to treat the patient, not the x-ray.

I had taken care of patients with HIV and AIDS before and I knew I could handle it. What I didn't know was whether I could handle Ava's attitude. After I reviewed his chart, I was ready to talk to him again and I was determined to do so. Without the mask, the gown, and the gloves, I knocked on the half-open glass door and invited myself in.

"Hi Ava, are you still nauseated?" I asked.

"Not you again, you don't know when to stop don't you?" he replied.

"Well, I just wanted to make sure you are comfortable," I said. "I can give you medication for your nausea if you would like, we don't have to wait for Dr. Ward's order you know." I continued.

"Ok, you do what you have to do," Ava responded with a voice that sounded a bit nicer.

I thought I should quit while I was doing well so I said goodbye and wrote a medication order on Ava's chart to help his nausea.

That evening, I was not on call so I got to go home and sleep in my own bed. After checking out with another intern, I headed straight home and into bed. There was practically no life other than the hospital when you are an ICU intern. You work, you go home exhausted, and you sleep and go back to the hospital the following day. This is exactly what I did the following morning. I made my rounds usually before seven o'clock in the morning and tried to write the notes before the attending physicians arrive at the unit.

There were five patients in the ICU when I left the night before but there were three new admissions, so overnight my patient load almost doubled. I was not going to visit Ava that day because, after all, he did not want any medical students or interns taking care of him. But when I got to the ICU, I was told that Ava had two seizure episodes overnight. Ava had an emergency CT scan and a neurologist was consulted.

I went downstairs to the Radiology department and before I could even look for Ava's films, Dr. Roberts, the radiologist called my attention. He knew about my interest in radiology and in fact, I had asked him to write a letter of reference on my behalf.

"I have an interesting CT scan here Bernie," he motioned for me to come over to where he was. The head scan showed small rounded masses on both sides of the brain. To make things worse, the masses were causing edema, a swelling reaction of the brain.

"What do you think is going on?" Dr. Roberts asked. I knew he was going to ask me that. He always asked me difficult questions and I really hated it at the time because I could not answer most of them, and that made me feel really stupid. But I got used to it. Looking back, I thought this was his way of teaching me.

"Contrast enhancing mass with edema in the brain, Ah…, it could be tumor or infection," I said.

"Well, which one of the two, make up your mind," Dr. Roberts said.

"Maybe tumor," I replied.

"Maybe is right," he said. Then he continued, "on a patient with AIDS, you can't tell if this is infection or brain tumor such as lymphoma, the best thing to do is to treat it like it is infection, do something for the brain swelling and then wait and see if it will go away."

I was fascinated on how Dr. Roberts just casually makes his diagnosis from the CT scan. After all, he was trained as a neuroradiologist and had been doing it for seven years. I was also impressed that he knew a lot about the patient, something unusual for a radiologist.

Then he asked, "Is he your patient?" Before saying another word, I looked at the Identifying name on the sheet of film. Above the date of the exam and the medical record number, it said Roger Stamp.

"Yes he is, he is my patient," I replied. After thanking Dr. Roberts, I went back to the ICU and resumed my rounds.

Having seen Ava's head CT scan, I went directly to ICU room number 3. To my surprise, Ava was already up sipping on broth for breakfast.

"Well good morning young doctor," Ava greeted me. I stood by the door in amazement because I thought he would be too sick to eat or even speak.

"The medicine you gave me really worked, I feel good today," he said.

"It's wonderful, I am glad it helped. But you're still not out of the loop you know. We still have to make sure that we are giving you the right antibiotics to take care of the bugs growing in your stomach," I explained.

"And my seizures?" he added.

"Well, we have to take care of that too," I quickly responded.

Ava smiled as if satisfied with my words of encouragement. I tried to change the topic because I did not know if I had the right to actually tell him about the CT scan results, he was a private patient of Dr. Ward after all.

I asked if I could listen to his chest. Sitting by the edge of the bed, he positioned himself turning his back towards me.

"Deep breaths please," I instructed as I positioned my stethoscope so that I could listen to both of his lungs while I watched his bony chest expand. His body looked worn and exhausted. Then I positioned my stethoscope on his chest and listened to his heart.

"Your heart and lungs sounds good," I said.

"That's great," he smiled as he replied.

I briefly examined his sad, sunken eyes and pale, dry skin, signs of dehydration due to fluid deficiency brought about by his constant vomiting and diarrhea.

"By the way, no one was here with you yesterday, would you like us to call any of your friends or family members?" I politely asked.

Ava smiled and then he said, "Honey, it is so sweet of you to ask but all my family members were out late partying last night and at 8:00 AM they, for sure, are still in bed." He continued, "You know I missed a show last night, I am a star you know."

"I am sorry to hear that," I said trying to sound casual as I wrote my findings on the medical chart.

"You don't believe me, do you?" He said.

Before I got a chance to respond, Ava started talking. "I am a performer, I am very popular you know, I sing, I dance, the total package. I do a great Barbara impersonation."

"Barbara Streisand?" I asked.

"But of course honey, is there another Barbara?" he said. I looked at his direction but chose not to comment. "There is no sense talking to you," he said sounding irritated.

"No, but I am sure once you have the make up on, plus the act and the attitude, I am sure you are very good," I said.

"Now we talking honey," he said laughing.

"Well, I am glad that you are feeling better and when Dr. Ward gets in, I am sure he will discuss the CT scan results with you," I said before I left.

After a couple of days, Ava's condition seemed to deteriorate. His seizures would become more frequent and the vomiting worse. He also appeared to get weaker and weaker. On one occasion, I spoke to Dr. Ward about Ava's prognosis being very poor and that he was to consider hospice care. I was not surprised with his health's rapid decline, I almost expected it knowing Ava's very low T cell count. But what bothered me most was the fact that Ava had been in the ICU for four days and nobody had visited him, no fans, no admirers, and none of his so-called friends. I am sure having AIDS already made him feel alone but he must have felt even worse not having family members or friends visiting him.

I looked at Ava's chart and tried to see if there was a contact number of any family member that I could call and inform about his condition. On one of his older charts, there was a contact person with an address and a telephone number. The chart was seven years old and I was not sure if the contact number was still valid. When I dialed the number, an older woman answered the phone.

"Hello, I am calling from the Hospital, and I am an ICU intern," I said.

"How can I help you?" A soft crackly old female voice responded.

I was nervous when she asked the question and I did not know how to start the conversation even though in my mind I had already practiced what to say.

"Are you Roger Stamp's mother?" I asked.

There was a long pause and then she said, "yes, yes I am."

I told the lady that her son was in the hospital for a serious condition but chose not to elaborate much. I was expecting that she would ask a barrage of questions but the only thing she asked was directions to the hospital and the room number.

A few hours later, an old couple showed up to the ICU and introduced themselves as Roger Stamp's parents. Ava's mother had a short curly white hair, her face much older than her age of sixty-two. She had on a pair of red pants and white blouse with no embroidery or design. The simplicity of her attire all the more brought focus to an embellishment pinned on the right side of her blouse, a rainbow broach. As she was talking to nurse Tina, she kept an indescribable facial expression, perhaps a combination of excitement, concern and sadness. Ava's father was short and a little on the heavy side. He was wearing a baseball hat, which he removed upon entering the ICU, exposing his hairless head, and heavily wrinkled forehead. Just like his wife, Ava's father also looked very concerned.

"I think he is sleeping," nurse Tina said as she accompanied them to Ava's room. When Tina left the room, the sliding glass door was shut but the curtain was halfway open and I could see what was going on inside the room from the nursing station. Ava's parents stood by the foot of the bed looking at their sleeping, bedridden son.

Not too long after, Ava woke up and tried to get up but was immediately stopped by his mother who then sat by his side. Ava's mother was crying as she ran her fingers thru Ava's face feeling every bony curve before she tightly embraced him. His father who was initially standing, frozen by the foot of the bed, moved closer and reached for Ava's hand. Ava appeared overwhelmed and tears started streaming down his cheeks, the very first time I ever saw him show true emotion. Once again, he tried to get up and prove that he was doing fine, but he was too weak to do so. It was one of the most moving images that I had ever witnessed, a scene too powerful to describe. After a few minutes, Dr. Ward arrived in the ICU and went directly to room number 3 when he was notified that Ava's parents were there.

I would usually join the attending consultants as they do

their ICU rounds, but at that time, I had chosen not to. I wanted to give the family their much-deserved privacy as they discussed treatment options with Dr. Ward.

The rest of the day went on without incident. I sent home three patients, and there were no new ICU admissions. It was the end of the month and was my last day in the ICU. The new intern should be pleased to start out with only four patients.

After checking the vital signs, making medication adjustments and finishing other paperwork, I made my final round to check on all the patients before I left for the day. There was a laboratory test result still on the printer so I checked it. It was a simple blood test that proved the patient was anemic and dehydrated. This was nothing new to the patient in room 3. As I took the laboratory sheets and placed it inside the chart, I saw an order on the physician's notes. It was a phone-in order from Dr. Ward, "DNR (do not resuscitate). I knew it will happen soon and I was not surprised. As I closed Ava's chart for the last time, it was then that I realized something different on the face of the thick, heavy plastic covering of his chart…the red sticker was no longer there.

THE DARKROOM

"Ask many of us who are disabled what we would like in life and you would be surprised how few would say, "Not to be disabled." We accept our limitations."

-        - Itzhak Perlman

Dawn was upset because for the third day in a row, she was again scheduled to work inside the "darkroom" developing x-rays. "I didn't go to x-ray tech school just to be cooped up inside this dark hole all day," she says cussing as she entered the small room carrying the cassettes of films containing the x-rays ready to be developed. Although she did not really slam the door, she closed it just hard enough to show her discontent. Even with the door closed, one could hear her feet's heavy steps, making noise as she opened the cassettes, took the x-ray films out and ran them into the processor for developing.

Outside the room, I stood by the bin from where the developed x-ray films emerge from the processor. I sometimes wait impatiently although I know that each film has to go through the entire developing process, soaked in various chemicals, washed and then dried before it comes out of the processor. Of course nowadays, a lot of x-ray departments utilize digital technology that is essentially filmless. Once x-rays are obtained, the digital image no longer needs to be processed. It is immediately ready for viewing and interpretation seconds after its acquisition. The data are sent to the reading station computer and made available to all authorized physicians who have the hospital computer access code.

The darkroom is strategically located in between the two x-ray rooms so that the x-ray cassettes can be easily moved and processed. Outside the darkroom is the tech area, perhaps one of the busiest places in the department. This is where the technologists hang out, wait, and check the films they took before they are brought to the radiologist. In essence the area outside the darkroom becomes the designated quality control area. But in the same way that it is a place of business, it is also a place to socialize, and a place where gossip thrives.

"What are you doing here? you're not supposed to be reading x-rays today." Mike, the senior resident says as he came back from lunch. He was always very business like and direct to the point. The kind of resident who would do his job, teach and explain things but did not socialize a lot.

"I am sorry, I thought I was supposed to be here," I responded.

I was called to check an important referral from the emergency room because Mike was not there. He had been showing up late and took longer lunch breaks since he became a senior resident. He would always find a good excuse saying, "I fell asleep in the library studying for the board exams." But neither the consultants nor we, the younger residents mind. A lot of senior residents usually slow down as they are about to graduate. It is almost expected. In fact someone even coined a term for it, "senioritis," the disease of the senior residents.

It was my day to interpret nuclear medicine imaging studies so I headed to the nuclear medicine department, which was on the first floor of the hospital building. The nuclear medicine department is always less busy. The images take longer to obtain and since the hospital had only one scanner, the technologist was always busier than the radiologist. There were not a lot of studies to interpret that day. There were a few renal (kidney) scans, a couple of liver scans, but majority of the studies were bone scans looking for evidence of trauma or tumor spread. Included in the pile of studies I read that afternoon was the bone scan of Frank Jacobs

Medium built Caucasian man at his late forties, Frank was our "darkroom" expert. He had been limping for the last week experiencing pain in the shin of his left leg so he had taken a few days off. Even with rest and doses of acetaminophen, the pain persisted so he decided to see a doctor who ordered an x-ray of his left leg as well as a bone scan. The technologists felt Frank's three-day absence. They argued and pointed fingers as to who would take on his responsibilities inside the dark room. To a few people, it might seem like a welcome change of pace. But to many, it is a long unending routine of opening and closing x-ray cassettes and developing x-ray films in a small hot and inadequately ventilated room, lit by the dim glow of a small red light bulb. To most people, the darkroom is a torture chamber. For the last three days, Dawn was handed the task for she was the newest technologist in the department. "It would be a good learning experience for you," said the chief technologist who disliked Dawn since the moment she was hired.

For Frank, working in the darkroom was not a big deal, in fact it suited him very well. He would come in with his portable radio and work his eight-hour shift without any complaint. He would stay inside the small room and would only come out to eat lunch or use the bathroom. For the most part, he worked with his radio on, listening either to radio talk shows or to stations playing music from the sixties. He enjoyed his job and was very proud of it. He was not an x-ray technologist and he did not even finish high school so he felt very fortunate to have the job, one that he had kept for the last ten years. To Frank, darkness was nothing new because it is the only thing he had known. He was born premature and received high oxygen therapy. As a result, both his eyes were affected with a complex eye disease, a condition called retinopathy of prematurity. At first his parents were optimistic that the condition would spontaneously improve as they were lead to believe, but unfortunately Frank's vision never recovered and he had since been blind.

There was a focal area of increased accumulation of the radiotracer (a substance injected into the patients vein in nuclear imaging studies) on Frank's left lower leg corresponding to his area of pain. Although non-specific, the finding worried me. I knew he also had x-rays taken that morning so I compared the bone scan with the x-rays. To my relief, the x-ray showed an intact bone without evidence of destruction. It showed however, mild thickening of the cortex, the outermost layer of the bone. I called Frank at home to ask him questions about the symptoms he felt. From our conversation, he denied a single event of trauma or fall. "It hurts most whenever I run," he said pointing out that he ran three times a week. Given the imaging findings along with his story, I told him that his pain was probably due to stress fracture from repetitive trauma. I advised him to rest, to refrain from running in the meantime, and to follow up with his primary care physician.

"That's quite a reassuring news," Frank said before he said goodbye and hang up.

On my way to work the following day, I was surprised to see Frank getting off the bus to go to work. I thought he would be on leave and take the opportunity to rest his injured leg, but then again three days of rest might have already done it. Parked on the street and interested, I watched how Frank managed to go to work each day. On his left shoulder was a bag in which he carried his portable radio and perhaps his lunch. In his right hand he held a long wand that guided him as he walked. Tapping his wand and feeling the ground before each step, Frank advanced from the bus stop to the corner of the street. As if by instinct or by feel, he crossed the street when the pedestrian sign "walk" was lit, along with the other people. I don't even know if the others realized that there was a blind man walking amongst them. Continuously feeling the earth with his wand, Frank made his way to the entrance of the hospital. After I parked my car and before going to the nuclear medicine department, I went upstairs to the second floor to check if Frank had made it to the x-ray department. I quietly stood outside the darkroom door and listened. It was not very long when I faintly heard the Beatles' song "I want to hold your hand" on the background, and I knew Frank had made it just fine.

As I continued my training as a radiology resident, I became more and more interested in teaching. I would collect x-rays and other imaging studies with interesting pathology and copy them so I could have it on the residents file, for easy access during teaching conferences. I would go inside the darkroom and copy the studies late at night when I am on-call in the hospital so as not to disrupt the normal workflow. Nowadays, the task of collecting important and interesting x-rays is a lot easier because you can always take a digital photo of the x-ray. For other hospitals with digital x-rays equipment, the images are simply copied on a disk.

One early afternoon, I copied a very important film while Frank was still at work.

"Good afternoon Dr. Bernie," Frank greeted me as he sat on the stool inside the dark room.

"How do you even know it's me?" I asked surprised since I hadn't said a word.

"I just know it's you," he replied with a grin on his face. "Let me help you with those x-rays you want copied, I will do it for you," he said.

I was quite amazed that he knew who I was but even more surprised that he knew what I was there for. Although I was hesitant, I handed him the few x-rays that I had. It was hard to get the x-rays copied perfectly for I could barely see the settings on the machine in the dark room, but I was sure it was even harder for him not seeing the machine settings at all. Politely, I just stood back and had him do it.

I watched him take out unexposed copy films from the rows of boxes inside the cabinet, then watched him carefully closed the box, making sure the cover was perfectly in place before he returned it. Feeling the edges of the copy film, he could tell which side was up and which side was down. He carefully approximated the x-ray and the copy films together, and placed them on the x-ray copier as he adjusted the intensity knob setting. Watching in amazement on how he effortlessly maneuvered himself in the room, I was even more surprised when every single copy came out perfectly looking just like the original x-ray.

From then on, I let Frank copy all the x-rays for my teaching file. Each time I brought him films to be duplicated, I would stay in the darkroom and chat with him. We would talk about many topics including the one from the morning radio talk show. He would give his opinion and then he would ask mine. We would talk about a lot of things including current events, sports, and music. He knew the lyrics to every Beatles and Elvis Presley's songs and he wasn't shy to sing along whenever one of them was playing.

I remember one time I talked to Frank about his being blind. I was surprised how candidly he talked about it without any bit of resentment. "It would be harder if I was born with vision and then lost it, but this is all I have known," he said.

Then I asked him, "Do you ever get tired of seeing nothing but black?"

He laughed before he answered to correct me, "It is nothing like that, not all black," he paused shortly, and continued, "I also see red, blue, yellow and all the other shades of color in between. I may see color in a different way than others, but in my world I see them the way they really are."

I took his answer and did not ask him to explain further but at that time, I wasn't really sure what he meant until I got to know him well enough.

Sometimes I would ask him to describe how he pictures something like a plant, or an animal or a thing. I wanted to get some idea of how he viewed things. I even asked him to describe other coworkers the way he "sees" them.

"She is a good looking woman in her fifties, she's always well-dressed, and always smiling showing her dimples," he said describing Barbara, the chief technologist.

"Dr. Billy Groves is of average size, has very fair complexion, he has receding hair and wears a mustache. He is probably in his early forties but he looks older, maybe because of stress," Frank described the radiology director. "Dr. Mike Saunders is tall and has heavy frame, he is always serious but he is nice when you talk to him," he said describing our senior resident.

It was amazing how he described each individual with such accuracy and detail. He even described things that I don't notice. "When you are born blind, you learn to use your other senses more effectively," he said. But thru all his descriptions about people, I never once caught him speak ill about anyone in the department. Maybe he chose not to say anything bad, or maybe he "sees" nothing bad.

One unusually slow afternoon, half of the residents including myself, were sent home early for there was little to do. It was just a little past four, when I was swiping my parking lot card and saw Frank walking to the bus stop to head home. Since I was not on-call and had nothing particularly important to do, I parked on the street and approached Frank to offer him a ride home.

"Dr. Bernie, it's nice to see you," Frank said. He never seized to amaze me whenever he called my name before I even say anything. He would sometimes tell me that he "saw" me eating in the cafeteria or that he "saw" me on the lobby talking to other doctors. I used to think my cologne gave him a clue, but he still recognized me whenever I don't use it. Maybe it's the sound of my steps, or maybe it is a blind man's intuition, something I don't possess and will never understand.

Frank lived not very far from my apartment, about a fifteen-minute car ride from the hospital. By bus however, it would have taken him thirty to forty-five minutes. With a few minutes spent walking and the wait for the bus, Frank probably made it home by five o'clock everyday. During the ride we had our usual conversation about music and politics but it was the first time he talked about his family. Frank married late when he was already in his forties to a woman he met through a mutual friend. His wife stays at home and takes care of their four-year-old daughter. "I look forward to coming home and see my family each day," he said with excitement in his voice.

From our conversations, it was apparent that he did things

other people with "normal" eyesight did. He went to church on Sundays with his wife and daughter, enjoyed late evening strolls in the park, ate out on occasion, and listened to audio books. I also learned that running was not just his hobby, but also his passion. A certain program allowed blind people to be paired up with people with normal vision who would serve as their running companion and coach. Through years of practice, he developed stamina and learned the course enough to compete. He said he had won some local races and once qualified for a national running Olympics for the blind. "I didn't win, but it was a great experience," he said with a big smile on his face as if he was reminiscing.

Although it was a short ride from the hospital to his house, it was refreshing to talk to him in a different environment other than the darkroom. He wanted to invite me in to meet his wife and daughter but I said maybe another time.

One busy morning while I was performing radiographic studies, the technologists were talking about a memo regarding an initiative to convert the current radiology department into a filmless department and that would mean switching from conventional x-ray machines to digital technology.

"It's about time, on busy days like today, digital would work best...you just take the x-rays and you're done," Barbara, the chief technologist said.

"I agree, our patient load is getting bigger each day and since they don't want to hire new techs, then maybe they should go digital soon," Dawn, the technologist said.

I bit my tongue and chose not to comment because I knew

Frank could hear the conversation and he may not have wanted to hear this one. A filmless digital system would mean: there would not be a need for x-ray developing, and there would not be a use for the darkroom. As a result, there might not be a need for Frank.

That afternoon when I brought x-rays to Frank for copying, he seemed a little somber and less animated. I was sure he had heard about the possible changes in the department. I tried to bring out topics that usually livened him up, but I was unsuccessful.

Then Frank asked me, "Doctor, you think they would get rid of me once they have the department converted into a filmless digital system?"

Frank had the right to be worried, this is a job he'd held for the last ten years, a job he had became very comfortable with. Through this job, he was able to provide for himself and his family. I actually anticipated him asking me this question but I really didn't know what to say. I may be a doctor, but I was a resident without any insight on administrative decisions that the department would make.

I looked at Frank, his head bowed down resting on both of his hands, obviously worried. The news had caught him off guard. Then I started to speak, "Frank, what you heard is true not only for this hospital but eventually for each and every radiology department. It is a sign of changing times and we can't help it. But nobody knows when this is going to happen." I paused a little bit to see his reaction but he kept silent. "I can tell you this," I continued, " If they decide to move forward, the process could take months and maybe even years, there is plenty of time to think on what your next step is going to be."

Frank lifted his head and said, "you're right doctor, I should not worry about it now, there is plenty of time, you're right."

I picked up the copied films looking like the original as usual. I thanked Frank and told him I'll catch up with him soon.

A few days later, I stopped by to say hi to Frank, just to see how he was doing. He was already back to his original self, animated, full of life and full of stories. We both never mentioned the proposed changes in the hospital again.

After the following months, the hospital got even busier with the radiology department getting more referrals. On my last day of residency in the hospital, I worked just as I would have any other day, saying goodbye to other physicians, nurses, techs and personnel throughout the day as I saw them. Fifteen minutes before four o'clock in the afternoon, I saw Frank sitting by the door outside the darkroom, he usually doesn't come out until a few minutes after four. I headed towards his direction and before I said anything he uttered, "Doctor, they kept you busy even on your last day."

By this time I was no longer surprised that he knew it was me. "What are you doing sitting out here," I asked.

"Well," he said and then briefly paused. "I don't want to miss the opportunity to thank you and say goodbye."

Looking at my watch, I felt bad because I was so busy to realize it was late in the afternoon. "I also want to thank you for all the help, for all the advice and the friendship," I said.

He stood up, set his wand by the door, walked towards me

and extended his right hand until it met my left shoulder. "You never asked me to describe you," he said.

I laughed before I said, "Well, I am afraid of what you're going to say."

His hand still on my shoulder he said, "You are a good looking young man, good looking inside and out." Then Frank reached for his wand, started tapping the ground and walked back inside the darkroom.

A few years later when I came back to the hospital to give a lecture, I was given a tour of the department by one of the younger residents. They had renovated the receiving area and added chairs. There is also new carpeting. The x-ray rooms had been repainted and they installed new machines. They had removed the darkroom making the tech area look a lot more spacious and less busy. Then I asked the resident, "Does Frank still work here?" His face went blank obviously he didn't know who Frank was. Barbara who happened to be there said that Frank had taken an early retirement, but then he went back to school.

I looked towards the direction where the darkroom once was. The same spot where I copied so many interesting pathological cases that I still keep up to this day only I had converted them into digital images for better storage. The darkroom to me was a refuge, an escape, and a classroom… Frank was the teacher and I was the student. In the darkroom, I learned a lot about medicine, about life, but most of all, it helped me see things the way they really are.

CHOICES

"Two roads diverged in a wood and I – I took the one less traveled by, and that has made all the difference."
- - Robert Frost

When I got to the hospital one morning, I was told that the surgeon had requested an invasive radiologic procedure on a three-year-old girl who had been admitted to the hospital just a little past midnight because of severe abdominal pain and fever. The patient's CT scan had been read by one of my colleagues on duty the night before. It only took me a short time to finish interpreting the x-rays from the emergency room because the radiologist on-call had already read many of them. I briefly reviewed the new patient's abdominal CT scan to have an idea on what I was dealing with before I headed to the short stay observation ward to talk to our patient and her family.

There was minor construction going on in the hospital by the stairs closest to the radiology department so I proceeded to the elevator. Rarely do I use the elevator to get to any other floors of the hospital, after all there are only five levels.

"Hold the door please," I said as I rushed towards a nearly packed elevator by the lobby.

The elevator was almost full and the occupants all seemed to know each other as they were all carrying on, talking and laughing. I squeezed myself in and attempted to press the fourth floor button but it was already lit, as were the second, the third and the fifth floors. The elevator stopped at second floor but nobody went out. The two teenage boys inside the elevator started laughing. The elevator then stopped at the third floor but again, nobody went out. The two boys burst into laughter once again, and then everybody started laughing. I figured they had just randomly pushed the button for all the floors just for the heck of it. I felt slightly out of place as I was the only person in the elevator who was not in on the joke and I felt quite uneasy. I could not wait to get out of the elevator. I felt a sigh of relief as the elevator stopped at the fourth floor but as soon as it opened, they rushed to get out and I was pushed to the side.

I headed towards the nurse's station and looked for the patient's chart. Michelle Hinkle, room 407 A, there it was on the chart bin. Abdominal abscess from ruptured appendicitis was the admitting diagnosis. This is a serious complication of appendicitis that needs immediate attention to prevent further spread of the infection. I proceeded to read the surgeon's notations that confirmed his request for the patient to undergo a CT scan-guided drainage of the abscess to be done by the radiologist. I checked the laboratory tests obtained early that morning to make sure they are within normal range for the procedure to continue.

I noticed that the anesthesiologist had already spoken to the patient and the family about the procedure.

Room 407 A, is a semiprivate room but the other bed was not occupied at that time. There were several people inside the room aside from Michelle who was lying on the hospital bed. I immediately recognized the two boys from the elevator. A middle-aged lady with strikingly red hair, neatly combed into a ponytail was sitting at the foot of Michelle's bed. There was a large, burly middle-aged man in rugged jeans and a checkered, long sleeve shirt standing at the head of the bed watching Michelle. There were several other people in the room, some of them sat on the empty bed and some occupied the chairs by the window. They were all familiar to me, the same people I had ridden in the elevator with.

I politely introduced myself, "Good morning, I am the radiologist." I got everybody's attention but nobody said a word so I continued. "I am the radiologist who will be performing the procedure on Michelle this afternoon." I walked towards the patient. Michelle was awake and stable but a little drowsy. She was given pain medication with sedative effect.

"Are you the assistant?" a voice questioned. It was Mr. Tom Hinkle, Michelle's father.

"No sir, I am the radiologist who will be doing it." I looked towards Mr. Hinkle's direction who seemed a little displeased by my response.

After a brief pause he said, "Well, is someone doing the procedure with you?"

I didn't know where his questions were leading, but I responded casually, "There will be a nurse and an x-ray technologist in the room to help me, and there will be an anesthesiologist to provide the sedation." There was complete silence in the room and for a second, I thought I had said something wrong.

"I came here to explain to you in detail what I plan to do," I said trying to break the awkward silence.

"I don't think I have consented to anything yet," Mr. Hinkle said in a commanding tone as he sat at the foot of the bed next to his wife and crossed his hands in front of his chest. I did not know how to respond to his comment so I decided to explain the procedure as I had planned.

"Dr. Farber, the surgeon has asked me to perform this procedure to drain the abscess from your daughter's belly. The abscess is what's making her sick."

Her father interrupted me, "Why can't she just have the surgery instead?"

I was not exactly sure what the reason was, but I started to feel uncomfortable. I was there to explain the procedure and to answer questions and that is what I intended to do.

"In the past, in situations like this, patients went directly to surgery to have the appendix removed and the abscess drained. But sometimes patients are too sick to undergo surgery right away. For some patients, having a catheter placed to drain the abdominal abscess works very well. Patients are given antibiotics so that the inflammation could subside and then have the scheduled surgery when the patient is better and then remove the diseased appendix." I have given this litany many times before and delivering it very convincingly is something I have mastered thru the years. Since

I got no reaction, I continued, "The procedure is done under CT scan guidance where the catheter can be precisely placed at our target area which is the abscess." Although everybody was looking at me, I was not particularly sure if they had understood what I said. All of a sudden, the two boys started laughing and instead of stopping the boys, the father also chuckled.

I looked at the direction of Michelle to see how she was doing and then I proceeded with a more detailed explanation of the procedure, describing the size of needles and catheters that I planned to use, the length of the procedure and the expected recovery. I think this was the longest time I spent with the family explaining about the procedure.

"Do you have any questions?" I asked but the father did not say anything. I must have covered every single aspect of the procedure.

Then for the first time I heard the mother said something, "when can she start eating?"

"As soon as she wakes up from the procedure, we will give her something to drink and we will advance her diet as she tolerates it," I said.

I was about to leave when the father asked, "How many of these sort of procedures have you done?"

I did not feel like I had to name a number so I just said, "I have done this procedure many times before."

At this point I was thinking that he probably thought I looked too young to be doing these procedures, I have gotten that comment before. He could also be nervous, I gathered that Michelle is his youngest and only daughter.

Since there were no more questions, I said goodbye and left the room. I had not gotten very far when I realized I had forgotten to have them sign the consent form. As I was coming back, I heard one of the boys trying to imitate my accent and finishing it off by saying what sounded like "ching, ching chong, chong, ching," as the other boy laughed.

Then I heard the father said, "Stop it." I thought he was teaching his kids to be respectful but then I could not believe what I heard him say next, "I don't trust that Jap." I did not mean to hear any of these and I was wondering if I should be glad that I heard the father's comment. They made fun of my thick accent but there is nothing I can do about that, I was not born in America. I was not born in China as the boys thought, nor Japan, which the father thought. But two things I knew for sure, that they were making fun of me, and that they didn't trust me. From the beginning, I had known the father did not like me but I had no idea that it was because I was of a different skin color. I had not faced this problem before, at least not knowingly. At that time, I had two choices, I could go back inside the room and confront them or just drop the procedure all together and have another radiologist do it.

Why should I even do this procedure, I questioned myself. Everything I do will be questioned. And if I make a mistake, I knew there would be a lawsuit. I called the surgeon with the intention of letting him know that I was not comfortable doing this procedure.

"Could you page Dr. Farber please," I asked the receptionist. The phone rang and Dr. Farber answered on the other line.

"Jeff, I want to talk to you about the patient with the ruptured appendicitis," I said.

"Are you done already?" Dr. Farber asked. The surgeons were used to me calling them when the procedure was completed.

"No I have not even started, I just got done talking to the family," I was saying when Dr. Farber interrupted me.

"O really, I am glad you met them. They live out on a farm a couple of hours from the city but they insisted their daughter come to our hospital. I have known this family for years, the father is a very skilled carpenter and I ask him to work for me sometimes. Take good care of them alright." Dr. Farber sounded like he was in a hurry as he always does.

I did not know how to respond to what he just said, and the words that came out of my mouth next was, "I will, I will take good care of Michelle."

"Now what's your question?" Dr. Farber asked.

"I just want to tell you we will be doing it this afternoon," I said before I hung up.

My plan of declining to do the procedure had been thwarted. So there I was, left without an option. I told the nurse that I had already spoken to the family and instructed her to have the consent form signed before the procedure.

Michelle was transported to the radiology department. I met her and her family in the corridor outside the CT scan room. "The waiting room will be on the other side of the hall," I said to them "the procedure could take thirty minutes to an hour and if it takes any longer than that, I will send someone to notify you."

"I would like to be in the room", the father said in a non-compromising tone.

"It will be a sterile procedure and it is best that we try to minimize the people inside the room," I explained.

I figured he would not be very happy about this, so I offered that he could be in the CT control area where he could at least see the procedure being performed through a glass window. This is something I usually offer to medical and nursing students who wanted to observe, but I thought this ought to appease him. The mother, the two boys, and the other relatives proceeded to the waiting room.

Michelle was transferred to the CT scan table and the anesthesiologist started to administer medicine to calm her and put her to sleep. I instructed Melanie, the CT technologist to perform the initial scans. I waited for the preliminary images to show up on the screen but nothing came out. We tried it the second time and again, no images could be seen. I could not show any frustration because the patient's father could see me inside the room and I didn't want him to have a clue that we were experiencing a machine malfunction. I could feel my palms sweat inside my sterile gloves.

"Can you shut the main power off and try it again," I told Melanie. We waited for a couple of minutes for the machine to reboot and initialize. Melanie started to scan and this time, we were able to generate images.

I have done this procedure many times before but that time, I felt like all my moves were being overly scrutinized. After reviewing the initial images, I marked the area of interest on the skin. After injecting a small amount of local anesthesia under the skin, I made a small incision. Shelly, the nurse handed me the multipurpose catheter drainage set. I had worked with Shelly and Melanie many times before in similar situations and they were both very good at anticipating what I needed for the procedure.

As I punctured the patient's skin with the catheter, I felt the resistance as I went through the muscular layer of the abdominal wall. Upon further advancing the apparatus, I felt a sudden release of tension. I knew my catheter tip was already in the abscess cavity. I aspirated as much fluid as I could and just like that, the procedure was almost over.

"This is what's making her sick," I held up a large syringe full of aspirated pus as I yelled out towards the father's direction. I drained almost a pint of abscess fluid from Michelle's small frame. The final CT scan images showed that the abscess was now completely gone.

After cleaning and applying a bandage to the small incision site, I collected a small sample of the aspirated fluid to be sent to the laboratory. I thanked the anesthesiologist, the nurse and the technologist and then left the procedure room. I called the father and walked with him to the waiting room so I could talk to the whole family. I told them that the procedure was over and it went very well. "She will be in the recovery room for an hour then she will be transported back to her room," I said. It was the first time that I did not hear any questions or comments from the entire family.

The following morning when I was going to check on Michelle, she was already sitting up and eating breakfast. Her vital signs were all stable and the most important thing was that she no longer had fever.

"So, Dr. Farber has already given the go signal for her to eat," I said.

Michelle looked at me and said, "I am so hungry I will finish all of this." Michelle picked a peace of bacon and shoved it into her mouth, making a mess as she does it.

Then the mother said, "She looked so much better today doctor, the procedure made all the difference, thank you very much." It was the most number of words I heard from the mother since I met her. The father was not around at the time. He and the boys had gone home the night before.

"If she does well without fever for two days, maybe she can go home the following day," I said.

"O, her father will be pleased," she responded.

As expected, Michelle got better and was sent home three days after the procedure. I gave Michelle a small brown teddy bear before she went home.

A few weeks later, our receptionist told me that I had a visitor. I did not think much about it because I always have a pharmaceutical representatives visiting once in a while introducing new equipment, or wanting to know how we like using the equipments they sold to us.

"Send them to my office," I said casually while finishing the pile of x-rays in front of me. I walked over to my office and to my surprise, found Michelle there with her Dad. She was wearing a pink dress with a large lace bow tied around her waist, her hair was pulled back in a ponytail and she was holding the teddy bear I had given her before she left the hospital.

"Well, look at you young lady, you look so pretty," I must have embarrassed her for she hid behind her father's leg.

"Good morning doctor," Mr. Hinkle said as he extended his hand.

I received the handshake warmly saying, "Good morning to you as well, I am glad you stopped by."

"Michelle said she wants to see her Doctor, we both want to see you." Mr. Hinkle's tone was far different from how I recalled.

"It sure is nice seeing her like this, active and healthy and O, so dolled up. Have a seat," I said. Mr. Hinkle smiled as he sat down while Michelle sat on her father's lap.

"Doctor, we want to thank you for everything you've done for her, she's our pride and joy you see." Mr. Hinkle's sounded very sincere.

"You are very welcome, glad to be of help," I said pleased, and at the same time, a little embarrassed.

"We would like to give you something," Mr. Hinkle said while getting something out of a brown paper bag and placing it on top of my desk. "This is for you."

It was a wooden miniature model of a CT scanner. The craftsmanship was superbly detailed, complete with the movable gantry table that could go in and out of the large donut hole just like the actual machine. I was really surprised.

"Thank you, thank you very much". Not knowing anything else to say, I continued, "I can use this to explain what a CT scanner is to patients a lot better, thank you very much," I said again.

As I was admiring the gift, I noticed Mr. Hinkle's face lit up with a smile like I had never seen it before and just like that, the animosity between the two of us melted away. He talked about his hobby of building things and he said he got the idea when I let him sat in and watched Michelle's procedure. It was a very nice visit, one that I will never forget.

Most days are good days at work but there are definitely days that can be challenging. Whenever I am faced with an awkward or even ugly situation, I know I usually have time to pause and think on how I would react. Occasionally I react badly, sometimes I react well, and sometimes I don't react at all. More importantly, I know I have the capacity to react in such a way that an ugly situation could be turned into something more positive, more productive or even fun. When I first heard Mr. Hinkle's racist remarks, I was really upset and I thought I had to choose between confronting him or not performing the procedure. I never realized that I had another choice: ignore the remark and go on with my job. I went on to perform the task to the best of my capability. It was not only my job, but also my responsibility, and perhaps the only way Michelle and her family could get to know me better.

Mr. Hinkle's gift comes in very handy as I explain CT scan to patients and their family members. But to me, it was more than that…it reminds me that there is always a better choice.

ANGELO CAN FLY

"It is the wounded oyster that lends itself with pearl."
-     - Ralph Waldo Emerson

Having been trained in the United States as a Pediatric Radiologist, I am fortunate to be mentored by some of the best in the field. There are many people who took their time and patiently taught me a lot of things. I always believed that the knowledge passed on to me would be wasted unless I pass it on to others. This belief led me back to my native country, the Philippines, to share my experiences and expertise in the field. Many Filipino Radiologists go abroad for additional training, I thought if I was to come back and teach, more people can benefit from the process including myself. I am not a prominent individual nor am I a well-decorated professor, but I have a powerful passion for teaching and for my profession. In the Philippines, I am based at a large teaching hospital in Manila, but I have visited several other hospitals whenever I get invited to give lectures and case discussions. On some occasions, I join other health care practitioners when they set out on medical missions providing free health assessment and treatment for the less fortunate. I recount an experience on one of my early visits.

It was a drizzly morning when we set out for the medical mission in Metro Manila not too far from the base hospital where we gathered and met. The entire mission group rode in two vans. Dr. Gomez, the Head of Pediatrics led the first van. A lady in her late fifties, she had recently cut down on her clinical practice but had become more active on resident education and civic action responsibilities. She was on the van along with Dr. Abby Sanchez, a senior resident who had made all the arrangements for the mission which included contacting different doctor's offices and pharmacies asking them to donate nearly-expired medicine that could no longer be sold. Abby was able to solicit three big boxes of medicine which were meticulously sorted by three younger residents who were also in the van.

The other van was the service vehicle of the hospital. Squeezed in between the boxes of medicine and the portable x-ray equipment were two technologists, a medical student, a second year radiology resident and myself. I was invited to join Dr. Gomez' van but I chose to be on the hospital van with the radiology resident who invited me on the mission.

The road which actually only had two lanes had now become a four lane road, although there was really no extra lane as the vehicles just tried to find an open spot in order to advance. The jeepneys fully packed with passengers are richly adorned painted with attractive colors but becomes such a nuisance for the jeepney drivers would stop whenever or wherever they want to pick-up passengers. The vehicles were so close to each other, one could almost hear the conversations going on in the next car.

"Is it always like this?" I asked Rey, the radiology resident who doubled as my tour guide. Some days, I feel like I had asked him more questions than he had asked me.

"This day is not particularly busy because some of the jeepney drivers are on strike protesting the constant oil price hike, you should see the traffic when its raining, it is even worse," Rey explained. I chose not to make a comment but I thought if the vehicles would just stay in their lanes, they would get to their destination much faster.

The medical student sat very quietly reviewing a pocket handbook on medication. He knew he would be stationed at the pharmacy. I tried to make conversation with him but his answers were brief and to the point. I have noticed this every time I speak to medical students. Rey told me not to get offended and explained that the students are just shy talking to senior consultants. "Its part of the culture," he said.

I used the rest of the trip to observe the sights and scenery. With the traffic moving so slowly, I could fully appreciate the surroundings. There were new and large upscale establishments along Quezon Boulevard, car dealerships, office buildings, large bookstores, fitness facilities, and restaurants. There were several restaurants next to each other one may wonder how they can all survive the competition. Although I remember seeing some of them before, a lot has changed since I left for the United States nearly twenty years ago.

Halfway to our destination, we passed along Espana street,

the busy university belt. The road became familiar especially when I saw the arch entranceway of the University of Santo Tomas where I spent my high school and college years. I spent eight years of my life passing through that arch built in 1618. The oldest Catholic university in Asia is also known to produce some of the most prominent physicians in the Philippines. The University certainly helped determine the direction I have chosen in life.

My mind was still reminiscing my days at the University when I noticed the scenery has changed, the traffic now even thicker almost at a stand still as we approached Quiapo church. I almost forgot it was a Friday, the day of the Holy Nazarene. Hundreds of devout Catholics, particularly the very poor and suffering make it a ritual to visit this church on Fridays. Just like the image of Jesus Christ carrying his cross, the devotees ask for blessing and help in carrying their own crosses. My sense of alienation having gone for so long was replaced by familiarity as I see the main street and along the narrowest alleyways close to the church, still lined with merchants selling herbal medicine and other concoctions. *"Gamut sa regla"*, a small bottle containing bark soaked in brownish-red liquid which was supposed to be good for relieving menstrual cramps looked the same as it did nearly twenty years ago. Those vendors also sell various types of dried leaves as remedies for cough and cold, high blood pressure, diabetes and other ailments. They also sell charms and potions that are suppose to ward off bad spirits. When I was a young boy, my mother would always stop by at one of these stalls after church service and looking back, it was as though the church was our hospital and the sidewalk our pharmacy.

Also visible pacing the streets were the children selling religious medallions along with the palm and tarot card readers. But Quiapo Church will not be without the *"sampaguita"* vendors. The small flower rosettes arranged into garlands that they sold exude a strong, sweet smell, temporarily masking the stench coming from the backed up drainage at the side of the church.

Not very far after passing the church, we arrived at our destination. The usual one-hour drive took two-and-a-half due to heavy traffic. The place announced itself as "Home for the desolate and unwanted children," as stated on the rusty metal gates. It is in the middle of a busy commercial district. The old building sits in a large compound surrounded with walls making the area almost a community of its own, a community of misfits I remember it referred to, when I was younger.

As we entered the gate, we could already see the nuns waiting in the lobby behind the large statue of St. Therese, their patron saint. I stretched my legs a little bit after getting off the van looking around the premises. I had been there before during a school-organized trip when we brought old clothes and canned goods. It was a memorable tour seeing the orphaned and unwanted children as well as kids with disabilities. I would have liked to have a quick tour of the facility to see the changes after so many years but due to time constraints, we planned to get to work right away.

They had set up two examination stations manned by the

pediatric residents to be supervised by Dr. Gomez. The donated medicines were organized on a long table just outside the rooms. Not all the patients got x-rays so when there were no films for interpretation, we helped the medical student and residents with the pharmacy. The drug manual listing the indications, dosages and contraindications of the medications came in very handy.

A room was assigned for us to set up our portable x-ray machine. One technologist operated the machine with the help of a volunteer nun. The other technologist converted the bathroom into a "darkroom" where he soaked the x-ray films on large plastic pails filled with developing chemicals and fixers before they were washed and hang dry. The x-rays were then brought to Rey and me for interpretation. The films took a long time to dry inside the bathroom so we decided to hang them on a clothesline by the garden. It made our waiting time a lot shorter.

There were a few skeletal x-rays for joint pain and trauma but most of the x-rays we took and interpreted that day were chest x-rays. The most common complaint was chronic cough suggesting possible tuberculosis infection. TB is an epidemic in the Philippines with higher incidence in people of lower socio-economic class. Our x-ray station did not have an overwhelming stream of patients unlike the examination stations so I was able to talk to the patients and get adequate problem history from the patients themselves.

One story was from a thirteen-year-old boy who had difficulty bending his right elbow. His x-ray revealed abnormal fusion and irregularity of the right elbow joint. In an adult, this could be caused by arthritis, previous infection, or even tumor. But for a young man, another possible cause would have to be post-injury. After talking to him, I found out that he sustained an injury two years ago when he jumped from the window of their burning house. His parents and younger sister all died during the fire. His fractured elbow needed surgical repair but he never had the opportunity so the bones of his elbow had now become distorted and abnormally fused that it would need a more complex surgical correction.

There was an eleven-year-old-girl who always complained of abdominal pain. Her x-ray showed four coins and a metal bolt in her abdomen. These metallic foreign objects were most likely in her intestines given their location on the x-ray. The nuns were also concerned that she had bald spots in her head, so I raised the possibility that she might have been pulling her hair and eating them too.

Another patient that I will always remember was a five-year-old boy labeled to have severe mental retardation. He had an unusually small head size for his age and had a crooked, rigid posture, that if his arms and legs did not get regular stretching exercises everyday, he would be spending his life in a fetal position. He also had "staring spells," that I believed to be seizures. The boy's problems had been present since birth but due to financial difficulty, the parents did not have the chance to seek medical care for their son. At two years old, the boy was left at the shelter. I knew that a CT scan or even an MRI would be the best imaging study for the boy's head but we did a skull x-ray anyway. To my surprise, we saw areas of calcification in the patient's brain. Given the clinical history and the x-ray findings, we raised the possibility of a developmental abnormality in the brain possibly from infection while the child was still in the mother's womb.

The number of patients had thinned down, and we thought we'd have no more films to read when Sister Grace brought me a chest x-ray to interpret. A lady in her late forties, Sister Grace is the administrator of the shelter. Although petite, she had a very distinguished posture and spoke eloquently that she commanded attention. After a brief exchange of pleasantries thanking us for our time and service, I focused on the x-ray.

Although the patient's name and date of birth was on the film, there was no medical history, and I had no idea why the film was obtained. Inspecting the film after hanging it on the view box, I observed that there was motion, poor positioning and substandard technique in taking the x-ray. It had been obtained from another institution two days ago as evidenced by the date sticker.

"This Kid is Angelo Romero, thanks for looking at his film," Sister Grace said in a loud happy tone. "He is a ten year old boy who returned to us five days ago, he had been coughing and we just wanted to make sure if he is okey," she continued.

Angelo already had a tuberculosis skin test, which turned out to be negative but the x-ray was obtained as a precautionary measure. He had his x-ray taken at an outside facility but they knew there would be a pediatric radiologist visiting so they kept the x-ray for a second opinion.

I turned my attention to the x-ray, inspecting the different shadows of the heart, the blood vessels and the lungs. I was about to interpret it as normal when I noticed the absence of the upper extremities. It looked like a real finding, the shoulder joint although small was present, but there are no arms, I thought to myself.

"So what do you think?" Sister Grace asked interrupting my thought process.

"The lungs look clear," I answered. Then I asked, "Does he have arms?"

Sister Grace, almost apologetic, said, "I am so sorry I forgot to tell you that Angelo is a Thalidomide child". It was then that I recalled from my remote memory that Thalidomide, a sedative used in the sixties can cause physical deformities in a child when taken by pregnant women. I knew the medication had long been banned and I had no idea as to how the mother got hold of the medicine, but I didn't bother to ask the question. Sister Grace did not only give the clinical history but also continued to give a brief summary of Angelo's life.

Angelo had been left at the side gate of the shelter one early morning ten years ago. "It was a dreary morning just like today," Sister Grace recounted. A beautiful happy baby with large smiling eyes and red cheeks, he was not even crying when the guard found him while doing his early morning inspection of the vicinity. He was comfortable and warm, wrapped in several layers of blanket. Everybody was wondering why such a beautiful baby would be left but this question was immediately answered as the layers of blanket came off when he was inspected.

My interest in Angelo's story would prompt sister Grace to tell me more about him. No one would adopt him because of his deformity. The people at the shelter knew him for who he was and he was not ridiculed. When he was three, an older couple adopted him but when his foster father died unexpectedly three years later, he was returned. A younger childless couple took him in when he was eight but it turned out they were not able to deal with the social pressure of having an armless child. Angelo ran away and managed to come back to the shelter. He pleaded that he be allowed to stay and call the shelter his home until such time he could be on his own.

Sister Grace knew so much detail about every resident in the shelter. Maybe because this was her responsibility as the administrator, to review and follow each resident's history and progress, maybe she needed the details whenever she met with donors, or maybe she needed them when she met with people for possible adoption. But in the short time that I had come to know Sister Grace, she made me feel as though she had a genuine desire to know each and every single resident because she wanted to, and because she cared for them. She talked about the residents with so much pride as if they were her own children.

The medical mission was successful. The group was very efficient finishing all the examinations just a little past noon. We were ushered into a room for a nice lunch reception prepared by the nuns and volunteers. The pediatric residents discussed the various cases they had encountered and exchanged medical opinions. I on the other hand was thinking about the most interesting x-ray I had read that day, the x-ray that we did not shoot and the only patient that I did not get to see. I approached Sister Grace and asked if I can meet Angelo. Without hesitation, she said yes.

The building housing the institution is shaped like a rectangle with the north portion of the building housing the administration offices and the multipurpose activity rooms where we had our medical stations. Across the courtyard on the south end of the building lie the chapel and a flower garden where they harvest roses for the altar offering. To the west side are the rooms for infants, young children and children with disabilities, and to the east are the rooms for older children and teenagers.

I thought Sister Grace would take me to the east wing of the building but we went to the west instead. Next to the activity center is a large room occupied by several metal cribs lined with a thin mattress. Although the white paint gives a clean appearance to the cribs, they were undoubtedly old. From the corridor, one can see everything inside the room through a glass window. The orphaned infants, age one to six months old would be in this region of the building until they get adopted or old enough to be transferred to another area. The next few rooms belonged to toddlers and young children. Each room housed four children. Adjacent to these rooms is a large play area where donated stuffed animals and other toys are available. Just beside the play area, is the section of the building that houses disabled children. Here, a community of children born with cerebral palsy, Down's syndome, and other abandoned children with physical and mental disability resides. The hall was built dormitory style with rooms on either side of the corridor. Several volunteer nursing and physical therapy students help take care of the residents. Angelo's room was at the very end of the hall, where he would remain isolated until his tuberculosis skin test and chest x-ray are both cleared.

The door to Angelo's room was slightly open and we could see him sitting by the window. He seemed busy doing something, his head was bent toward the floor where several sheets of paper were scattered.

"Angelo, you have a visitor," Sister Grace said as she knocked on the already opened door.

"Please come in," the boy said politely as he gathered the sheets of paper with his feet to put them away. I was about to help him but to my amazement, he was quick to use his feet, the way I would use my hands. I didn't know how to greet him, I usually extend a handshake whenever I meet people including children, but of course it would be inappropriate in that situation.

"How are you doing," I asked. The boy stared at me as if assessing my purpose for the visit.

"If you are here to take me away, forget it, you are wasting your time," the boy's demeanor changed as he put the papers on his lap and adjusted himself on the chair to look away from me.

Sister Grace intervened, "Angelo, he's the Doctor who looked at your x-ray, he just wants to meet you."

After a brief silence, the boy looked at Sister Grace and said, "I'm sorry."

The nun approached the boy and gave him a hug to reassure him everything was fine.

"Do you want to listen to my heart?" the boy said pointing at the stethoscope hanging around my neck. As a Radiologist, I rarely used a stethoscope but I kept it with me that day in case I had to examine patients.

"O yes, of course I do," I said as I approached the boy, placing the stethoscope on his back and listened to his lungs. I then placed the stethoscope on his chest and listened to his heart. As I listened to the boy's regular heartbeat, I had a closer look at the sheets of paper on the boy's lap.

"His heart and lungs sound clear sister," I said to Sister Grace. "Those are very good," I said referring to the papers the boy had been working on.

"O those, he drew them you know, Angelo likes to draw," there was a happy tone on the nun's voice proudly talking about the boy's talent.

They were pencil drawings, sketches of children playing ball, running around having fun. "This is Toto, this is Isko, and that's David," the boy pointed out the characters on the paper. He had other sketches but most of them depicted children playing. The sketches had been drawn with such precision and detail that they looked almost alive on paper. I had to remind myself that those were sketches drawn by a ten-year-old using his feet.

"These are great drawings, you are a very talented boy," I said going thru the pieces of paper. Angelo smiled and seemed to enjoy the complement.

When Sister Grace left the room to answer a phone call, I asked Angelo why he was not in any of his drawings. "Those kids were playing, I was just watching," the boy said. I sensed a bit of sadness on his face. "I just watch, they never asked me to play with them," he continued. Other than the absence of his arms, Angelo appeared to be in very good physical health and obviously very capable of things, but maybe other people see it differently.

"Maybe they think you don't want to play," I said.

"Or maybe they don't think I can play, maybe they think I can't do what they do," the boy answered quickly.

I did not know how to respond to what he just said. At that point, I knew I had in front of me a boy who is not only talented, but also smarter than a lot of the other kids I knew.

As minutes passed talking, the unfamiliarity between Angelo and me vanished. I listened to him tell me stories about a lot of things. He told me how he likes ice cream and cake and how he looked forward to the end of each month when they served them at the shelter. He also talked about his favorite television shows, and how he preferred game shows better than cartoons or *telenovelas*. Then he said he likes the shelter, and how he wished he would live there forever. He talked about his friends and Sister Grace but not once did he mention his previous foster parents so I did not bring up the topic.

After I felt I had gained his trust, I had the courage to ask him a question, "how do you feel about having no arms?"

He answered casually, "I don't know, I am used to it. I am used to people staring at me." Then he paused as if giving the question a second thought, "but I am sad, because people say I can't do a lot of stuff, you know, I'm different." I felt the little boy's comment like a stab wound; I couldn't even imagine how bad he must've felt.

I told Angelo that when I was a kid, I was really skinny and I got sick a lot. The other kids didn't want to play with me because they didn't think I was fast enough or good enough. Then I told him that since then, I tried hard to eat well and sleep early so I would gain weight and get stronger. I also told him that even for me who had both arms, things were not always easy. Angelo appeared to be listening but I was not sure if he truly understood what I was telling him.

"Close your eyes," I told Angelo. "Think about what you want to do right now, then imagine yourself doing it," I continued.

The boy hesitated but closed his eyes and I could tell that he was really concentrating.

After a few seconds, I asked him, "Tell me what you see."

Angelo's eyes were tightly shut but his face was lit up with a wonderful smile showing the deep-seated dimples on both of his cheeks. Then he said, "I am by the beach running very fast and I am flying."

I wasn't quite sure how Angelo was able to fly in his imagination, but his expression was enough to make me believe that he could really do it.

"I see you guys are having fun in here," the nun said as she entered the room, interrupting our conversation. Then Sister Grace told me the medical team was already looking for me.

"You can do whatever you put your mind into." I said as I stood up and gently ruffled Angelo's hair just before I left the room. I told him to keep in touch and I would do the same.

That night I thought about the boy, his disability, his wit and his talent. It amazed me that the person who had made the most significant impact on me during the mission was someone

I almost did not get to meet. Though I met with administrators, doctors and other professionals during my trip, it was this little boy who lived in a shelter of the desolate and unwanted who had shared the most, and taught me the most.

Weeks later when I got back to America, I received a package from the Philippines. The address was that of the homeless shelter that I visited. The envelope was heavily cushioned and had a "do not fold" label on it. I was sure it was a thank you note along with a copy of brochures about the shelter, something I requested so I can distribute it to people I know. Sandwiched in between two pieces of brown cardboards was a charcoal painting.

The strokes on the drawing were so delicately done that despite the single color used, the scenery looked so alive, giving an illusion that it was colored. In it, Angelo was by the beach playing with his friends. His face was wonderfully lit with a smile and obviously having fun. His feet were slightly lifted off the ground as his playmates looked in amazement. In the drawing, he had no arms but he had wings spread widely outstretched getting ready to fly.

I paused for a second and absorbed the beauty and meaning of the sketch. This must have been the scene going thru his mind when I had asked him to close his eyes and imagine what he wanted to do. There was no letter attached, not a simple note or dedication, but at the bottom right corner of the sketch, it simply read, "Angelo can fly".

A Child's Battle

"A physician is obligated to consider more than a diseased organ, more even than the whole man, he must view the man in his own world."

-      - Harvey Cushing

I had just gotten into the hospital and put down my briefcase when I heard the loud cry and scream of a young child resonating in the radiology department. Following this noise led me to the computed tomography suite that at the time had more people than usual. Consultants, residents, medical students, nurses and technologists, a room full of unfamiliar faces alternately consoling a screaming child probably does not help ease that child's agitation.

Entering the room, I set the adjustable light switch knob to low, a trick an old mentor used whenever he tried to pacify a screaming child. I tried to do the same on selected patients and although it sometimes does not work, it has almost become a habit. But on this patient who had nothing to eat or drink for the last eight hours in preparation for a procedure, nothing would probably work better than a sedative.

Dr. Diaz was the anesthesiologist that day. She was one of the more senior anesthesiologists, and was usually the one assigned to administer sedations on severely ill patients and children having imaging studies in the radiology department. It was always difficult to predict how she was going to give her medications but that day, everyone knew that oral sedatives would not work.

"Let's start an I.V." She said as she opened her medication box and reached out for a twenty-gauge needle. She thought a bigger needle would be better for faster flow of the contrast dye in her veins. Just as when the child had momentarily calmed down, perhaps from exhaustion, the sight of the needle again made her hysterical.

It took four people to hold the patient down, a nurse, two radiology residents and myself, just to get a vein access for the medication. Using every bit of energy she had, the girl screamed, swung her arms, tried to kick and almost managed to lift herself from the CT table. Who would have taught that a frail and chronically ill little girl would have such strength? The hospital gown she was wearing came undone exposing her protruberant abdomen. Everyone was so relieved when Dr. Diaz was able to get the needle into a vein on the patient's right hand, and not too long after the sedative was injected, the girl took one big breath, yawned, and then started snoring.

Kristy Castro was the name printed on the hospital band tied around the child's right wrist. She was three years old but her appearance was more like that of a two year old or even less. Her name didn't sound familiar, I told myself. No one had spoken to me about the patient before the examination. Usually, the radiology residents notified me whenever there are pediatric patients scheduled for CT scan procedures.

While the resident was fixing the child's hospital gown, it was hard to ignore the child's overly distended abdomen, and around her belly button, there were many prominent blood vessels that resembled a disorganized spider web. Her skin, so dry and scaly had a yellowish hue that matched her jaundiced eyes.

Now that Kristy was already sleeping, everyone stepped outside the CT suite except for Dr. Diaz who wanted to stay inside the suite to monitor her patient. "Don't worry about me, I've had enough kids and they are all grown up, you can radiate my ovaries anytime," the aging anesthesiologist said so casually that it was hard to figure out if she was joking or not. But I still gave her a lead apron to help shield her from radiation during the procedure.

Separated from the CT suite by a leaded glass window, we gathered at the control station. I took the first available chair to watch the scan being performed. I opened the patient's medical chart that was lying on top of the console table only to find that the thick plastic folder contained so many pages of disorganized loose papers that trying to make some sense of it was nearly impossible. The patient had recently been transferred from another hospital that did not have any imaging facilities other than conventional x-rays. They sent a photocopy of the patient's entire chart but someone must have dropped it on the floor and now the pages were all mixed up.

Painfully going through the mess of paperwork, I was lucky to find a half-page discharge summary. It was short and incomplete and did not contain the course of treatment or plan of action at the other hospital, but nonetheless, it was very helpful. It stated the working diagnosis as "end-stage liver disease," confirming my suspicion. Unfortunately, it also said "etiology unknown" meaning no one had figured out what had caused the girl's liver damage. I quickly checked the laboratory values for the liver functions but it offered no additional information.

"Give me the possible etiologies for end stage liver disease on our patient," I asked the residents hovering around me not pointing to anyone in particular. The awkward silence was broken by a senior radiology resident who started the discussion on "infections such as hepatitis." Following him, one by one the remaining residents enumerated other possible causes including congenital diseases or others inborn errors of metabolism, biliary problems, medication-induced or other non-specific inflammatory processes. A medical student said alcohol can cause liver disease but it was immediately pointed out to him that the three-year old patient probably had never ingested even a drop of alcohol. Then someone brought up the subject of prognosis and just before I answered this question, I noticed a man quietly standing in the corner of the room. He did not look familiar to me, and he was not wearing scrubs or a white coat so I was sure he was not a technologist or a physician in training. He wore a plain white shirt and faded jeans. His stocky appearance and golden brown complexion made me think he was a working man who spent a lot of time under the sun.

I got up and extended my hand into a handshake and introduced myself to the man.

He in turn introduced himself, "My name is Delfin Castro." He was the patient's father. Unlike most parents who would immediately ask what I could see, Mr. Castro just stood there and waited for us to do what we needed to do. I did not even realize that he had been there standing throughout all our discussions and I wonder how he had felt listening to us talk about his daughter's illness. For a moment, I was a little worried that we might have mentioned something that had alarmed him.

"The images are ready," said Ruben, the CT technologist. Much like the radiology system we used in the United States, my host hospital in the Philippines, known as one of the best hospitals in the world, also uses the same filmless system. After every examination, the images are sent to the viewing station and the study is read directly from the computer monitors. I told the residents to review the study so that we could discuss it later. Meantime, Kristy was transported to the recovery room for observation, a practice not routine for all the post-sedation patients but due to the child's ailments, special precautions were being taken. At that point, I offered to accompany Delfin to the waiting room.

"I am just so glad we got this study done Doc, we have been waiting for so long," Delfin was almost ecstatic, clenching both of his fists as if he had won the lottery. At the back of my mind, I was thinking, this should have been done three years ago but I kept my mouth shut.

"You from the States, right Doc?" he asked just to start a conversation.

"Yes I am," I replied.

"You know we have been in and out of the hospitals both in the Ilocos province and here in Manila, we almost gave up," Delfin said.

As we walked, it was obvious that Delfin was admiring the hospital, looking at the shiny marble floors, the fancy furnishings and the ivory colored walls adorned with paintings of famous Filipino artists.

"I hesitated when a stranger told us to come to this hospital about our problem, I know we couldn't afford it," he said.

One of the best in the world, the hospital catered to the elite, the wealthy and powerful members of society, but they do have social services department that helps cover hospitalization and treatment of selected indigent patients. Although the tests and hospitalization are not entirely free, there is a substantial discount.

"Kristy had all sorts of tests and they were all taken cared off, in fact this is the last study, maybe we can finally find out the cause of my daughter's illness," he said.

Suddenly, I felt a huge responsibility knowing that the man in front of me and maybe the referring physicians were relying heavily on CT examination results for the diagnosis.

The recovery room waiting area was empty. It was very different from the radiology reception area in which at least ten people were waiting at any given time. Delfin sat down on the comfortable leather couch. I was about to leave when Delfin started talking about Kristy, when she was born, when she was growing up, and her illness. Not very long, I myself sunk into the comfortable couch listening to Delfin as he recounted his only daughter's battle.

Kristy Castro was born a little over three years ago in an impoverished town of Ilocos Norte. The first and only child of Delfin and Nelia, Kristy got all the love and attention any child deserves. She had been born healthy they thought with two arms and two legs, crying when hungry and sleeping afterwards. Almost immediately though, Nelia noticed a slight yellowish color to Kristy and she did express her concern but the elders said it was common and would soon go away. Often, Nelia would wrap little Kristy in light clothes and they would both sit outside the house to savor the morning sun, something the town nurse told them would improve the baby's condition. But after days and even weeks, Kristy's unusual color would not get better, instead it became more apparent. After several doctor's visits, series of blood tests and an ultrasound of the abdomen, the provincial doctors told them that Kristy had a liver disease. Already saddened by the news, the young couple was even more puzzled because the doctors would not give them an explanation as to what caused their daughter's condition.

The young couple lived with Delfin's parents, and owned not much property or possessions other than their clothes in the dresser. Delfin made a living making charcoal. Once a week along with another man, he would go into the forest collecting sticks and twigs that they would bring back to town using the *"kariton,"* a cart with wheels entirely made out of wooden scraps.

The dried out pieces of wood they collected were placed inside a pit in the ground and are ignited with the flame and heat kept to a minimum so that the wood carbonizes and turns into charcoal. The day Kristy was born, the flames were not monitored and the entire week's hard work turned into ashes.

Nelia worked in a tobacco factory, hand-rolling the tobacco leaves layer by layer keeping them tight and straight, a skill she learned from her mother who did the same job before she passed on. Nelia continued working until late into her pregnancy but since her daughter's birth, she had stayed at home. Although she wanted to work, her child's ailment prevented her from doing so.

I sat there and listened to Delfin talk as if he had known me for a long time. For a moment there, I realized he probably was so overwhelmed that he just wanted someone to listen to him and I just happened to be there. I would intermittently say "yes," "aha," "Oh, really," but for the most part I just listened.

Once in a while they would go see a medical specialist in Manila, an eight-hour bus ride from their province. But later on, their trip would become more and more frequent so it was more convenient for them to stay in Manila. The Castros decided to move so they could be closer to a Children's hospital and get better care at least for emergency reasons until they found out what was really wrong with Kristy. They were fortunate enough that Nelia's aunt invited them to live in their house without paying rent. Delfin looked for a job and was immediately hired as a garment factory worker. The pay was minimal but it helped sustain his struggling family and at the same time he could pay a small part of the rent at least to share in the electric consumption and other utilities.

"It's difficult to accept that our only child has a severe liver disease," Delfin said before he let a long sigh as he shook his head. In his eyes one can see a combination of disbelief and despair. Then he continued, "We went to see other doctors for a second opinion but they all said the same thing, end stage liver disease of unknown etiology." The big reality was that Kristy had a severe and incurable disease.

In the CT reading room, the residents had already looked at Kristy's examination images when I got back. "So what do you guys see?" I asked after I quickly reviewed the images. Rico, the senior resident confidently enumerated his findings. "Kathy's protruberant belly is due to her large and mottled liver floating in significant amount of free fluid within her abdomen. The veins around the liver are dilated and backed up suggesting a long standing disease." Rico is one of the brighter residents but this time he forgot to mention another finding. Pointing out the prominent tubular structures along the esophagus, I explained. "These are dilated veins called varices, it is important to note this finding because it could be a cause of hemorrhage in patients with chronic liver disease." The examination clearly depicted the primary disease along with the secondary complications but was not specific as to the cause of the liver problem. Despite the advances in CT technology, there are still things that cannot be answered and which would definitely need correlation with laboratory findings or even a specimen sample of the liver itself.

Since I was the radiologist who reviewed Kristy's CT scan,

I was invited to attend the treatment management conference that day. It was ten minutes pass one o'clock when Rico and I headed for the conference room. I felt bad about coming in late but as we entered the room, I was surprised to find out that no one else was in the room other than Dr. Solomon, the pediatric resident taking care of Kristy who was reviewing his powerpoint slides. Looking preoccupied and tense, he would be presenting the patient's clinical history.

It was a small but well equipped conference room, the type one would use for meetings rather than lectures. In the center of the room is a large, neatly lacquered rectangular table made of *"kamagong"* wood. The well-cushioned chairs surrounding the large table have leather upholstery. A digital projector was secured on the ceiling facing the large white screen at the north end of the room. Rico and I sat at the end of the table closest to the door so we could easily excuse ourselves should we get called for an urgent reading or procedure in the radiology department.

Not long after we sat down, the gastroenterologist arrived and sat across from us on the table. We exchanged greetings but she later resumed to review the patient records. A few minutes later, more people came in. One by one, physicians in long white coats entered the room. Although the names and faces of the physicians were not familiar to me, I could tell the department they represent, inscribed just below the right lapel of their white coat, "Gastroenterology and Hepatology, Pediatrics, Surgery, Pathology..." One could recognize that most of them are senior consultants because they had blue identification badges. There were only very few residents and no medical students. At this point, it was apparent to me that this would not be a regular teaching conference.

Dr. Solomon presented Kristy' clinical history from birth to present highlighting her hospitalizations, clinical and laboratory test results. The pathologist was called upon to describe the findings from the liver biopsy performed a couple of days ago. I then showed and discussed the findings on the CT scan: the enlarged liver, the abnormal free fluid, the dilated veins both in the abdomen and extending into her chest. Everyone paid attention. I had no idea how many physicians in the room had already seen the patient but at least the CT examination gave them tangible images that they could easily correlate with the laboratory findings. After I spoke, the gastroenterologist summarized the important facts in determining the patient management strategy.

Finally, the surgeon made the announcement everyone knew was coming: "So there is no question about it, this child needs a liver transplant." He said. "In fact with all the clinical data presented, this patient will have no chance to live a longer life without it," he continued. Many people inside the room who agreed that Kristy's only chance to survive is a liver transplant echoed the surgeon's sentiments.

"The surgery as well as the post-operative care carries the possibility of complications. Can the patient handle all of these; is she healthy enough to manage all of these?" A very important point was brought up by one of the physicians standing at the back of the room. There were many more physicians who came in filling the small room.

"Although we know she has extensive liver damage, we still

don't know what caused it. How sure are we that the transplanted liver will not fail again?" a pediatrician spoke pointing out another important fact. The comment incited other thoughts; "Maybe we can't do anything," said one. "Maybe it's too late to do anything," said the other.

There were several more questions asked: about certain laboratory tests, about the transplant donor waiting time, and about the surgery itself. Having met Kristy's father Delfin, I was aware of the family's living standards and financial situation. I shyly raised my hand to speak, "Getting the transplant, waiting for a donor, the surgery itself and the long process of post-operative care, hospital and doctor's visits, laboratory tests and medications, who will pay for all of these?" I was not very familiar with the hospital's policies and I knew that the expense from all of these would come with a huge tag price, one that the Castros would not even start to comprehend. I was relieved when someone from the social services department spoke that a huge amount had been allocated for hospital's charity work and that if the decision is to push through, the hospital will shoulder the majority of the financial burden. Still, the Castro's would have to come up with a substantial amount of money.

Then someone raised an important point, "Why not use that money for children who will have a better prognosis, someone who is very sick but has a better chance of long term survival?" The comment brought the room to a brief silence, and although no one said anything in support, no one in the room disagreed.

Although it was obvious that the child would not survive

without the liver transplant, what was not clear was: Does Kristy deserve a chance to undergo a liver transpant?

The meeting lasted nearly three hours. The patient, the family, the transplant management team, the facility and the financial resources, many important issues were brought up and taken into account. At one point, there was even a heated discussion between the transplant surgeon, the allergologist, and the intensivist. It was interesting to have witnessed the deliberation process.

Though difficult, the group eventually arrived at some sort of consensus: a go signal for a liver transplant.

I stood up and introduced myself to some of the physicians in the room but immediately went back to the department to finish reading the pile of x-ray films that have accumulated in the meantime.

More x-rays, more decisions to make; which ones are normal, which ones are abnormal. The job so routine to me yet in every single film or study, I think, I deliberate, I decide. It is not everyday that I get to participate in the decision process on whether a patient gets a liver transplant or not and I don't even know if this is a privilege. Yet on a small or large scale, I get to make decisions that could impact someone's health and life, this I take with a full sense of responsibility.

It was ten minutes before six o'clock when most of the pediatric studies had been interpreted and I walked to the parking area to head home. Aunt Glo's canteen by the parking lot was now closed, there were fewer cars parked, and the cigarette vendor had already left; all signs of a working day coming to an end. Comfortably anchored in the car seat before I turned the ignition on, I saw Delfin sitting at the small picnic area by the parking lot. Not far from him is a young lady blowing bubbles in the air. That must be Nelia, I thought to myself. Then I saw a young girl, her gait wobbly trying to run despite the weight imposed by her enlarged liver and retained fluid in her body. Oblivious to her pain and illness, you can see her try to reach for the bubbles in the air, just as any child would, she would try to catch every single one of them until it bursts and vanish in the air. Oblivious to her illness, the little girl seemed to be having fun, laughing as she tried to run. After all, this life of sickness is the only life she knew, the same kind of life both Delfin and Nelia has become accustomed to.

It was a very loud, unrelenting cry that signaled the start of my workday but it had ended with an image of a laughing, happy and well-loved child. The irony was, it had the same source, a fragile, dying, three-year old child.

It was already early evening when I turned the ignition on and got ready to head home. It was peak time for the evening traffic, with noise and confusion ruling the streets as I drove off. Despite the chaotic background around me, I felt a comfortable calm. That day more than any other day, I was sure about my chosen vocation.

EMMANUEL'S GIFTS

It is our duty to remember at all times and anew that medicine is not only a science but also the art of letting our own individuality interest with the individuality of the patient.

> \- Albert Shweitzer

One afternoon, I received a call from Dr. Jonathan Van Knapp, an obstetrics and gynecology physician. At the age of thirty-five, he was the youngest among six obstetricians in the hospital but had the busiest practice because of his reputation as a smart and hardworking doctor with good bedside manner. He was also known for his excellent skills and knowledge on ultrasound that very rarely did he call upon the radiologist for a second opinion. He even had several arguments with the other radiologists in my group contesting what he thought to be inaccurate ultrasound interpretations. A few times when he needed my opinion, he would only show the printed images for review. But on that day, he kept the patient in the room and wanted me to repeat the ultrasound examination.

"Please take a look at the patient in room C," Dr. Van Knapp said. He never referred typical or ordinary cases and I knew it wasn't going to be easy.

I headed for the OB department, a newly renovated annex, which was conveniently connected to the pediatric ward of the main hospital via a skywalk. This made it easier to transport sick infants especially during winter months. After swiping my badge through an automated card reader, the double door opened and I entered the new center for the first time since its renovation. The new building had a fresh atmosphere brought to life by the vibrant baby blue painted walls complemented by pastel colored furniture and decor. There was still residual smell of paint, which was far more pleasing compared to the distinct yet unexplainable odor of amniotic fluid that used to fill the air inside the old OB ward. Letters of the alphabet designated the rooms rather than numbers, and each room functioned as the delivery room, recovery room, and nursery, all in one. The new annex was given the name: The Birthing Center.

By the door outside examination room C, I saw Dr. Van Knapp wearing surgical hat and scrubs, which was his typical attire. A surgical mask still hangs around his neck as if he had just finished a C-section. He was talking to Drs. Gary and Lynn Phelps, a married couple who are both pediatricians. Their voices were low but one could tell that they were engaged in a serious discussion. I had no idea why a pediatrician would be consulted on the case because as far as I knew, the patient was only six months pregnant and was not in active labor. I politely waved my hand to introduce my presence as I passed them, but I was careful not to interrupt their discussion and went directly to the nurse's station to review the patient's medical records.

I picked up the medical chart of the patient in room C that belonged to a certain Stella Domingo, a single, 23-year old, Hispanic female. Stella was six months pregnant and presented to the hospital complaining of vaginal bleeding and abdominal pain for two days. Her OB history stated that she was G3 P1, which meant that she had been pregnant three times but delivered only once in the past. I initially thought this was a mistake until I later read that she had a previous abortion. Her medical and social history was quite complicated but was extensively documented by the medical student in three handwritten pages. From the chart, I gathered that Stella had a longtime battle with alcohol and substance abuse. She was also in and out of prison for various petty crimes and parole violations. It was in prison that they found out Stella was pregnant when they subjected her to undergo a urine pregnancy test following a fainting spell and episodes of vomiting. She was still on probation for shoplifting and public intoxication but was released to the care of "Heaven's door," a residential shelter for unwed and homeless women. I sorted through the other useful information on the chart including blood work and other laboratory tests that she had before I returned her chart back onto the nurse's desk. As I was walking back to the ward, I saw Dr. Van Knapp once again who stopped me at the hall.

"I don't have a good feeling about this one," he said while shaking his head.

I was not sure if he was referring to Stella or her unborn child but I didn't bother to ask.

"Don't worry, I will do a thorough ultrasound examination," I said.

He stood closer to me, placed his hand on my shoulder, and whispered, "you better do a good job, Gary and Lynn would be adopting the child."

I was happy to hear the news about the adoption, but I was worried because Dr. Van Knapp's facial expression was more of dismay rather than excitement. I asked Dr. Van Knapp where Gary and Lynn were but he just shrugged his shoulders before he walked towards the nearest phone, and rushed to answer what seemed to be an important page.

Gary, Lynn and I graduated from the same medical school. We spent many hours together for we were in the same group in Biochemistry and Physiology classes. We also spent countless days together studying and dissecting cadaver in Anatomy class. Through the years, I had come to know both of them not only as colleagues but also as friends.

Gary is a man of few words and an over-all nice guy who had always done things by the book. Before going to medical school, Gary used to be a Physics professor but he resented the fact that a lot of his students did not take Physics as seriously as he did. He left teaching, took the medical college admissions test (MCAT), and passed it without any difficulty. He was very knowledgeable but at the age of 35 when he started medical school, he was the oldest in our class and had found it challenging to keep up with his classmates who were at least ten years younger. Gary and

Lynn started dating during medical school and got married after graduation when he was 38 and she was 34.

Lynn left her mother in Vietnam when she was only nine years old to live with her biological father in America. Lynn's father, a former GI had another family in the United States who welcomed and treated her as a true member of the family. Through the years, she kept in touch with her biological mother in Vietnam but the lady she called "mom" was his father's wife. Being half American and half Vietnamese, she said she always felt odd and out of place so she always worked extremely hard to prove herself and be noticed. "Nothing comes easy for me, I work hard for everything I have," I remember she told me way back in medical school.

I had known about the Phelps great desire to have a baby, even resorting to in-vitro fertilization twice. The delicate and expensive procedure called for Lynn's egg cells to be harvested from her ovary, had them fertilized by Gary's sperm outside the human body, and implanted back to Lynn's uterus. The first time they had it, the pregnancy did not happen. On their second attempt, the pregnancy progressed and at one month of gestation, ultrasound documented three fetuses with active heartbeats. The notion of having triplets excited the couple, but a follow up ultrasound a month later showed only one fetus thriving. Disappointed but still very hopeful, Lynn stayed home and made sure she did everything right to preserve the pregnancy. Not long after, she experienced severe bleeding that signaled the fetus' demise.

When I entered room C, a thin middle-aged lady with a short, curly brown hair greeted me. I thought she was the patient's mother but she introduced herself. "I am Marina, Stella's friend and social worker," she said.

"Good morning, please have a seat," I greeted her back. I approached Stella who was comfortably lying down and in no apparent distress. She had a rounded face that was even more emphasized by her short neck and shoulder length, black hair. Her upper body and pelvis were well covered up with blankets but her pregnant belly was exposed. There was a device strapped around her abdomen like a loose belt, which was attached to a machine that monitored her baby's heartbeat.

"How are you young lady?" I asked.

"I am good doctor, just a little nervous," Stella replied with an awkward smile that exposed the wide gaps in between her teeth. I also noticed a metal piercing through her tongue that gave her a little slur when she spoke. I was glad that she was not in active labor because a restless pregnant woman screaming in pain would be much harder to perform an ultrasound on.

I pulled the ultrasound machine closer to the head of the bed and adjusted the machine's viewing monitor so that I could easily see it. I also pressed the appropriate settings on the machine before I sat down on a stool right next to Stella's bed, and positioned myself for the examination. After I had readjusted the blankets around her pelvic area making sure I kept it well covered, I picked the appropriate *transducer* and squirted a water-based gel that would help maintain its contact with her skin as I perform the ultrasound.

"This is going to be cold," I cautioned her as I squirted more gel onto her belly. I spread the gel using the *transducer*, avoiding the fetal heartbeat monitor that was strapped around her abdomen.

"So this is your third pregnancy, is that right?" I asked. Stella answered me with a nod, which I took for a yes.

"So how were your other pregnancies?" I followed up with another question not meaning to be nosy, but I wanted to know if there were any abnormal medical conditions associated with her two previous pregnancies. Stella appeared nervous as she continuously tapped her fingers on the bed but Marina reached for her hand and squeezed it lightly which seemed to help a little.

"My first pregnancy was fine, it was a baby girl. That was more than three years ago, I gave up custody and she lives with her father now." She said.

Before I had the chance to ask about her second pregnancy, Stella looked at me and said. "I had my second pregnancy terminated." Her tone was one of confidence as if she was sure she did the right thing but the expression on her face revealed some sadness. "But this one's going to be different, I know, I can feel it." She said feeling the sides of her enlarged belly.

"No more gangs, drugs or alcohol. I am going to find me a job after I deliver this baby. I mean it this time." She said as she turned her head towards Marina, herself also a recovering alcoholic but sober for the last seven years.

Then Stella asked Marina, "Do you think I made the right decision to give up this baby?" Marina did not respond. She knew about Stella's lifestyle and although she did not express it, she knew that adoption would be best for Stella and her unborn child.

I have always tried to make conversation while scanning to put the patient at ease. This worked very well with Stella as she opened up and told me a lot of things about herself. I would ask one question, but she would respond with paragraphs. From our conversation, I learned about her life as an alcohol and drug abuser, how she was disowned by her family, how she survived being homeless sleeping in parks and shelters, and how getting in line at the local soup kitchen was a daily routine. We also talked about the adoption process and how she got to know the Phelps.

She was already three months pregnant when she tested positive for a urine pregnancy test in prison. At the time of her release, she had been sober for a month and had a clear mind to think. It was at that time when she decided to give up her unborn child for adoption. With Marina's help, Stella used the Internet to search for adoption agencies. She sorted thru a list of orphanages and institutions taking care of abandoned children until they narrowed the search down to agencies where pregnant women can give up their unborn child for adoption. Stella said she initially had plenty of families to choose from, but when her profile was sent to the prospective families, many of them backed out and only four remained interested. Stella knew that her child would have a better life if raised by any of these four families but after a long deliberation, she chose Gary and Lynn Phelps, both physicians who lived in Dayton, Ohio. By this time, Stella was already four months in her pregnancy and the only prenatal examination she had was a urine pregnancy test. She was urged by friends to go to the public health clinic but she never got around to do so.

The Phelps had been very supportive of Stella. They visited her, provided encouragement, took her out to dinner, movies, and even shopped for her. Stella said that the last two months had been great…she was sober and living the life she had always wanted. She had a roof over her head and food was always available. With Lynn's prompting, Stella eventually had a prenatal work up and laboratory tests but refused to have an ultrasound done because she didn't want to see an image of the baby for fear of developing an emotional attachment. Although disappointed, Gary and Lynn Phelps respected Stella's decision.

Our conversation was cut short when Dr. Van Knapp entered the room. Along with him is an OB resident, and two interns who seemed to have been clued in regarding the interesting case. The room became very quiet that one could almost hear the ultrasound probe as I glided through Stella's skin. Stella was also quiet, her face glued to the ultrasound monitor, almost mesmerized with what she was seeing on the screen. Marina squeezed Stella's hand, this time a little harder perhaps to calm herself rather than calm Stella. I proceeded to scan towards the pelvic area where the baby's head was positioned, looked at it on different angles and stored several representative images for documentation.

As I grabbed a clean piece of washcloth to wipe the extra gel off Stella's belly and replaced the *transducer* back to its holder, the inevitable question came. "What did you see, doctor?" Stella asked. At that time, I could not hold back. I had to tell her and everyone else in the room what I saw.

"It is a baby boy," I said to start, but this news did not generate any response from Stella nor to anyone else in the room. They were waiting for more. Then I proceeded, "the baby is not normal, the baby's brain is not well formed."

Stella responded to my surprise, "Well, we have a three more months to go, it will grow some more wouldn't it?"

After a moment of pause, I said, "It is not like that, much of the brain is replaced by fluid, a condition called *hydranencephaly*. The brain may have been normal at one time but an infection or other trauma to the child's brain has occurred. It is like your child had a massive stroke inside your womb." I could not have made the explanation any simpler but as expected, Stella had one question after another. No one else in the room dared to participate in the discussion. I had been in situations similar to this and I knew that there was no amount of explanation that would suffice. Then I proceeded to summarize, "The baby is alive but has a severe brain defect and his chances of long survival after delivery is very low."

Her head to the side with eyes fixed to the monitor showing the image of her unborn child, tears started to flow from Stella's eyes. Marina tried to comfort her but there was nothing that would comfort her at that time.

After the procedure, people left the room one by one…the interns, the OB resident, Dr. Van Knapp, Marina and myself. We all gave Stella some time to herself, which she requested. I went to the nurse's station and wrote a preliminary report on Stella's medical chart before I left the building.

On my way back to the radiology department, I saw Dr. Lynn Phelps. She seemed in a hurry and I didn't think she noticed me as we passed each other in the hall. She was carrying a fruit basket on her right hand and held a wonderful arrangement of fresh cut flowers on her left hand. Her hair was pulled back and the happy and excited facial expression on her face was easily recognizable. I wasn't sure if someone had already told her about the ultrasound result, but I was hesitant to tell her since it wasn't her who consulted me for the study. When I decided I would tell her, the automatic double door behind me had already closed.

All of a sudden, questions filled my mind. How would Gary and Lynn feel about the ultrasound results? Would they go thru with the adoption process? They have suffered enough and maybe they would just accept the fact that they can't have children. And how about Stella, how would all of these affect her? How long would the baby live after delivery? For sure this sudden turn of events would bring pain to a lot of people involved.

In the following weeks, I had not seen Lynn, but I spoke to Gary twice, each time I avoided bringing up the topic and which he also did. Having been around them for a long time, I knew how private they both were and if they wanted some help or advice, I knew they would ask.

Two months later, in early December, we got a request for a brain MRI examination on a newborn. The request simply stated; evaluate for congenital brain abnormality. This was something we dealt with on a fairly regular occasion but what caught my attention was the patient's name, which was listed as Baby boy Phelps on the request form. Right away, I had a feeling that I knew the baby, and I was right…it was Stella's child. The baby was born a month premature and soon after delivery, he was transferred to the Neonatal Unit of Hospital for further clinical and imaging evaluation. Since the baby's last name was Phelps, I assumed that the adoption process was carried out with both Gary and Lynn Phelps as the adopted parents.

Although the patient was awake and breathing, he did not move very much and we decided not to sedate the patient for the procedure. Multiple MRI sequences were planned but after I saw the initial images that showed a brain that was largely replaced by cerebrospinal fluid (brain and spine fluid), I instructed the technologist to just do one other sequence to shorten the procedure. After all, the diagnosis was already evident. The MRI study was confirmatory of my initial ultrasound report of *hydranencephaly*.

I knew that someone would be at the waiting area expecting a preliminary result, so I proceeded to the waiting area and found that Gary Phelps was there. He received the news as if he had already expected it and asked no further questions about the MRI. I asked him what his plan was and he said they would take the baby home as soon as possible knowing that there was really nothing that the doctors at the hospital could do.

Before he left, he handed me an envelope. "It was an invitation for our child's baptism and also our Christmas get together," Gary said as he helped push his baby's bed thru the halls and back to the hospital room.

It was December 19, a very cold Sunday afternoon and a snowfall was expected for that evening. I intended to go to church for the baptism but I was on call at the hospital so I wasn't able to make it. Instead, I proceeded directly to the Phelps' residence for the Christmas get together.

Their house was located in a suburb just south of Dayton. I parked on the street outside their house but for a few seconds, I hesitated because there was not another car on the street, which was quite unusual for a party. Then I thought that people were probably still at church. When I rang the bell, Gary opened the door.

"We have been waiting for you," Gary said, who seemed delighted to see me. He ushered me in and offered to take my coat to hang it in the closet. As we walked toward the living room, I noticed a very festive atmosphere in their house. This was something new because I always knew them as minimalists who were not really fond of excessive decorations. We passed a richly adorned Christmas tree and sat in a comfortable sofa next to the fireplace. While Gary was opening a bottle of wine, Lynn entered the living room. She had an apron on but underneath, she was wearing a red and green sweater that I had given her the previous year.

"We're so happy you could come, you are family you know?" Lynn's comment made me even more at ease. There was something new about her; she seemed glowing and contented, which was quite remarkable despite what she and Gary were going through. She had the biggest smile on her face, and after she gave me a hug, she pinched both of my cheeks, the same way she always did back in medical school. She sat and visited for a while but she had to go back to the kitchen and finish setting the table.

Soon after, an older lady entered the room. Her, silver gray colored hair was tied up in a bun that accentuated her almond-shaped eyes. She was wearing a traditional red and gold-colored Vietnamese dress made out of silk which covered her entire body. She was carrying the baby, which she cautiously laid in the crib by the living room.

"This is my mother in law Kim," Gary introduced her. I extended my hand, which the lady acknowledged. Lynn's mom had just recently arrived from Vietnam and although she understood English, she did not speak it fluently. She responded by a nod or by acting out pleasant gestures.

Then I approached the crib and focused on the baby.

"His name...Emmanuel," said the old Lady. The baby was comfortably sleeping just like any baby who had just recently been fed. I played with his tiny fingers but was careful not to wake him up. Although his eyes were closed, he had that calm and happy baby look. Just by looking at him, no one would suspect that he had a severe brain defect and that he had not much time to live.

A few moments later, the doorbell rang and Lynn opened the door, it was Stella and Marina. Marina looked the same, but Stella looked so much different. She had cut her hair short and had lost a lot of weight. Stella looked healthier and much happier. After a short exchange of pleasantries, they rushed to see the baby, which was understandable. I gave them space to visit and in the meantime, I walked around the house.

Not long after, Lynn had announced that dinner is ready. We all sat down on the rich and festively adorned table with the finest China and silverware. There was turkey, ham, stuffing, cranberries, freshly baked bread and my favorite sweet potato soufflé topped with caramelized sugar and almonds. It was indeed a feast.

After saying grace, Gary stood up raising his glass.

"May I propose a toast, this is for our son Emmanuel who had brought us so much blessings this year." Gary looked at everyone on the table sincerely acknowledging us for our presence. He also mentioned how happy they were to finally have Lynn's mother join them for Christmas for the very first time. After mentioning everybody's name, he paused to look at his wife before he made an announcement.

"We are expecting another baby, my wife Lynn is pregnant," Gary hugged his teary eyed wife.

"Here is to Emmanuel"

"Cheers"

I was sitting across the large window able to see the winter wonderland developing outside with soft flakes of snow playing with the wind before it touches the ground. As we raised our wineglasses to toast, I was struck by the beauty of the occasion and I really felt very happy for everyone. Emmanuel brought joy, strengthened relationships, and brought new life. Indeed, Emmanuel brought a lot of good things to everyone on the table including myself.

ACKNOWLEDGEMENTS

To God, I thank you for all the blessings that come my way. I will continue to share these blessings to others in your honor.

To my parents Crispin and Epifania, my sister Malou, brother Jun, brother Ferdie and his wife Lorna, my nieces Kristina and Robin, and my nephew Joshua. Your love, support, trust, and tolerance have been the source of my strength and inspiration to go on with life's adventures. To cousins Nelson and Velmor, niece Gwyneth, and my staff Janet and Gina, my sincere thanks for taking good care of me, making my life more comfortable and less complicated so I can focus on my work each day.

To all my mentors in radiology both in the USA and Philippines especially Marilyn Goske, Janet Strife, Lane Donnelly, John Racadio, Janet Reid, Stewart Morrison, Dave Cavanaugh, Fran Unger, Beth Ey, Mary Greene, Beth Kline-Fath, Anne Calkins, Barbara Wolfson, Dawn Light, James Weiss, Jack Farrell, Jim Clark, Vic Gregory, Bill Meyers, Dan Schultz, Jeff Benseler, Hahl Stahl, Joe Staab, Todd Brack, Scott Harron, Mark Sturgill, and Joe Lee. Thanks for all the wisdom and guidance you have shared.

To Nathan Concepcion, Nanette Goco, Sonya Dy, Raymond Piedad, Marvin Bautista, Maricar Paguia, Khristin Pulido, and Julius Ding, thank you for the friendship. I applaud your courage to continue what we have started.

To my superiors Mr. Joe Ledesma, Dr. Joven Cuanang, Dr. Edgardo Cortez, Mr. Raffy Solis, Mr. Nat de Vera, Ms. Marilen Lagniton, Ms. Edith Simeon, Dr. Filipinas Natividad, Dr. Butch Asis and Dr. Bobby Ramos, thank you for believing in my abilities and for your continued support.

Thanks to Mr. Gerry Los Banos and his wife Dr. Florence Villorente Los Banos for their suggestions and help in editing this book.

To all my relatives both in the Philippines and abroad in particular, the Layas, Faders, Dancils, Custodios, and Edios, and to all my friends and co-workers who continue to support and listen…my sincere thanks.